Say Goodbye to Back Pain!

Exercise, Nutrition, and More!

by Dr. Tiffany T. Butler

DORRANCE
PUBLISHING CO
EST. 1920
PITTSBURGH, PENNSYLVANIA 15238

Dorrance Publishing Co
585 Alpha Drive
Suite 103
Pittsburgh, PA 15238
Visit our website at *www.dorrancebookstore.com*

ISBN: 978-1-4809-2971-5
eISBN: 978-1-4809-2350-8

For my prince, Joshua. You have brought laughter, joy, and happiness into my life.

For my parents, Annie and the late William J. Butler Sr., for your words of wisdom, support, and continuous love.

For my siblings, Cheryl, Sherbie, William Jr., Crystal, and Lisa. Your personalities are unmatched.
I love you all!

Contents

Phase V: Preventing Back Pain at Home

Phase VI: The Importance of Physical Fitness

Phase VII: Eating for Recovery

Phase VIII: You Deserve a Pain-Free Life

Phase IX: Making the Change

Introduction

"He who cures a disease may be the skillfullest, but he that prevents it is the safest physician."
Thomas Fuller

I love this quote by Thomas Fuller. I believe prevention of illness or disease can save you time, money and energy in the long run. Through proper training, education and instruction, we all can learn how to better live our lives. I often tell people I exercise and eat nutritious foods because my body needs it and craves it. It is what my body loves. Sometimes, I too slip up every now and then, but I get right back on track.

The purpose of this book is to provide the reader with the necessary information to manage and treat neck and back pain at home. The main goal is to help those individuals who do not have access to healthcare, who cannot afford healthcare, who cannot afford doctors' visit (e.g. co-payments), who suffer from chronic neck or back pain, and who lack the proper guidance for managing neck and back pain.

Remember to take care of your body, it is a precious vessel and should be treated with respect. When you take care of your body, your body will take care of you. Your personal health should be a priority. When you are healthy, you can better serve yourself and others. Take responsibility for your health. If you don't like the current health state you are in, change it. Begin today, do something about it. Don't wait until tomorrow or next week, or until you finally get that gym membership. A new life begins today, right now.

I hope that you benefit greatly from the information written herein. Yours in health,

Tiffany T. Butler, D.C.

Phase I

Suffered an Injury, Now What?

You are more likely to injure yourself when you are fatigued.

Introduction to Phase I Living in the age of technology we have an advantage of discovering things with the stroke of a key. The Internet is not only used as a tool for the enjoyment of posting pictures and keeping up with friends, but it is a wonderful resource for information. Information that can be accessed twenty-four hours a day, seven days a week in a matter of milliseconds from anywhere in the world. Although most people will spend hours on the computer, watching cats behave like humans, they do not utilize time to explore ways to improve their lives. This chapter will give you a basic understanding of the anatomy of the back and what to do if you suffer an injury.

Chapter 1

Anatomy of the Back

"When a muscle contracts, it knows no direction; it simply shortens." Lippert

Back Muscles and How They Work

Have you ever seen an elderly person who is bent over their walker? Did you wonder what caused them to be in this stooped position? Eliminating those individuals who may suffer from degenerative disc disease (DDD) or spinal arthritis, which can lead to this hunched back position, however, weakened back muscles can be the cause. Poor posture can be a result of lack of exercise, your occupation (performing repetitive motions in awkward body positions), and weaken back muscles.

Skeletal muscles are the most abundant tissue in the human body. They are mainly located in the neck and back region, as well as the upper and lower extremities. These muscles work constantly to maintain posture by keeping your body in an upright position and moving your body through various body positions.

Extrinsic (Superficial) Back Muscles connect your trunk (torso) to the upper extremity and are involved with movement of the shoulder joint. This is the first layer of muscle visible when the skin and fat is removed from the back. See Table 1.1 for their functions.

- Trapezius
- Rhomboid (major and minor)
- Levator scapulae
- Latissimus dorsi

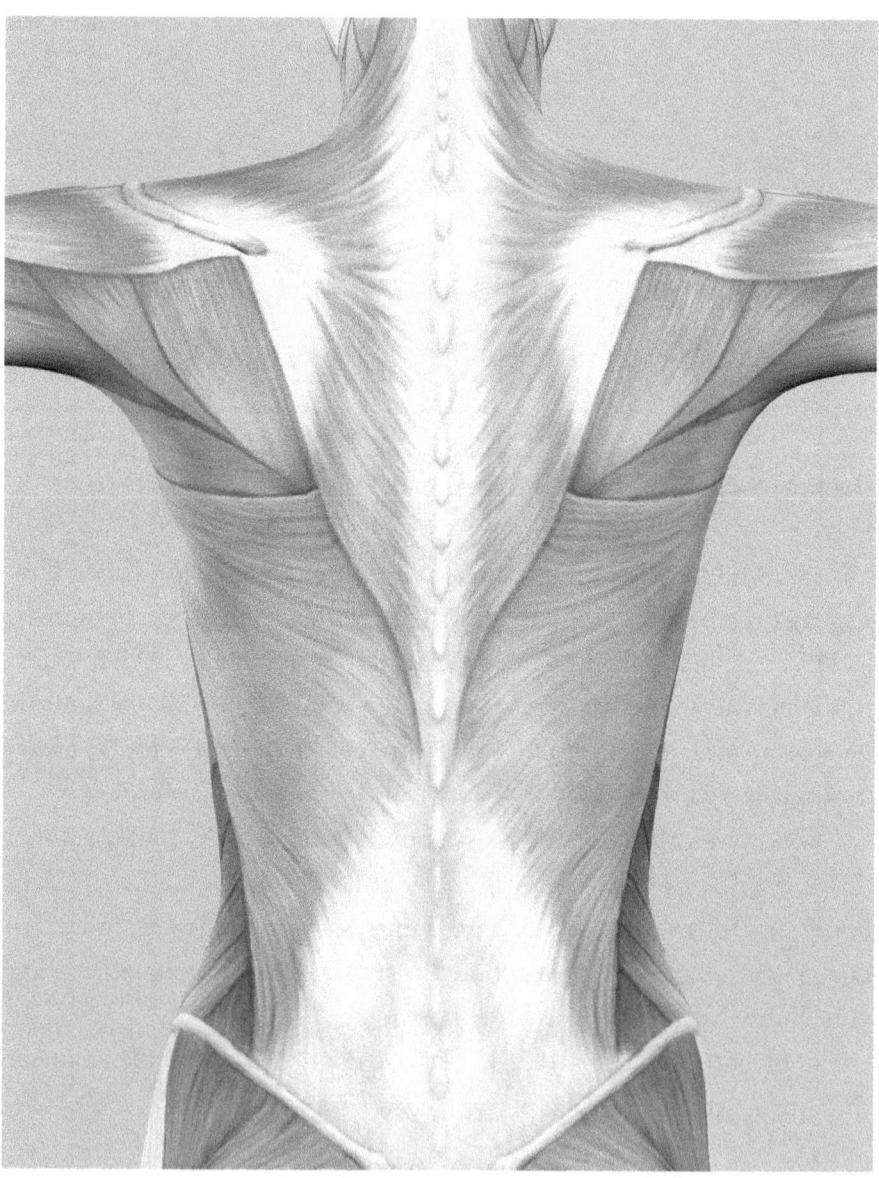

Table 1.1 Extrinsic (Superficial) Back Muscles	
Muscle	**Function**
Trapezius	• Movement and stabilization of the scapulae (shoulder blade).
Rhomboid (major and minor)	• Retraction of the scapulae.
Levator scapulae	• Elevate the scapulae. • Cervical rotation and flexion
Latissimus dorsi	• Movement of the shoulder joint (extension, adduction and transverse extension, in other words bringing your hand to your back pocket). • Extension and lateral flexion of the lumbar spine.

Intrinsic (Deep) Back Muscles extend from the back of the skull to the posterior pelvis and is involved with maintaining posture and movement of the spinal column. These muscles are most commonly injured by improper lifting techniques (such as lifting a box from the floor without bending your knees). See Table 1.2 for their functions.

- Splenius capitis
- Splenius cervicis
- Erector Spinae (Iliocostalis, Longissimus, and Spinalis)
- Semispinalis (capitis, cervicis, dorsi)
- Multifidus
- Rotatores

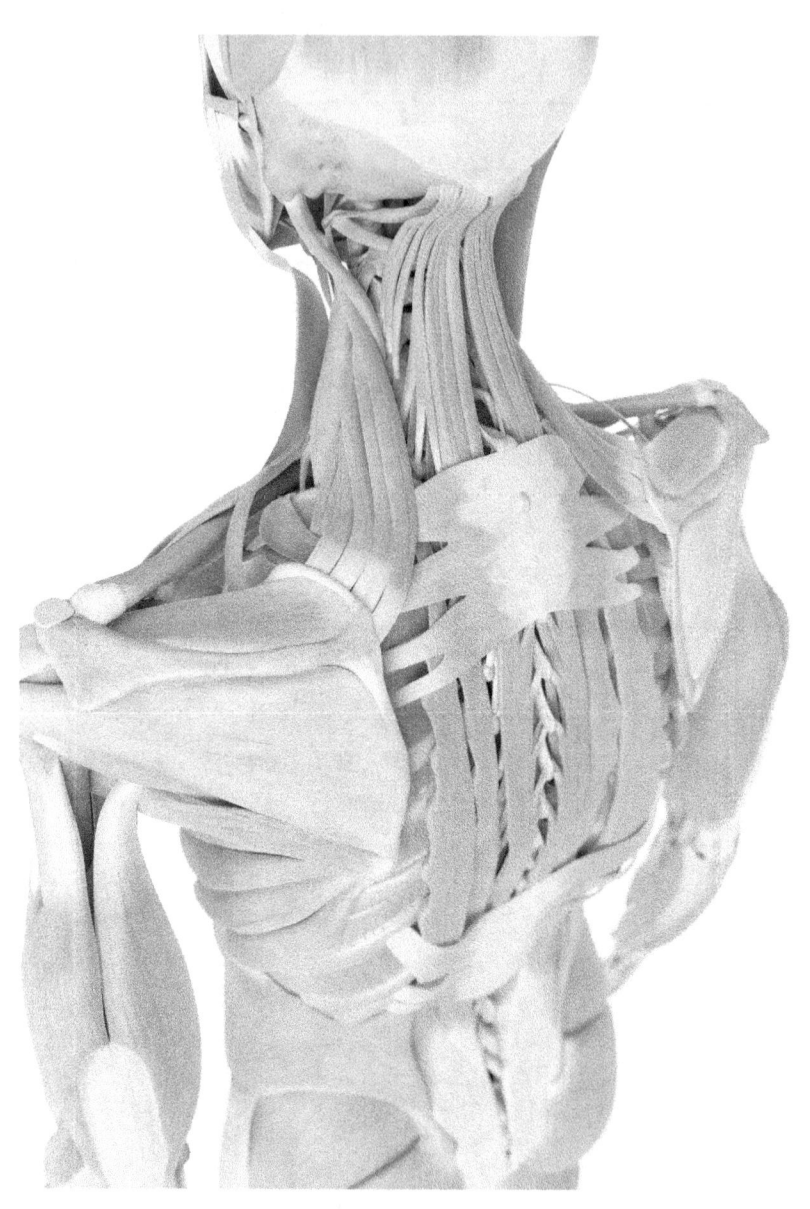

Table 1.2 Intrinsic (Deep) Back Muscles

Muscle	Function
Splenius capitis	• Head extension • Lateral flexion and rotation of the cervical spine.
Splenius cervicis	• Cervical spine extension. • Rotation and lateral flexion to the same side
Iliocostalis	• Extend vertebral column. • Flex head and neck to same side.
Longissimus	• Extend vertebral column. • Flex head and neck to same side.
Spinalis	• Extend vertebral column. • Flex head and neck to same side.
Semispinalis	• Stabilize vertebral column. • Extend vertebral column
Multifidus	• Stabilize vertebral column.
Rotatores	• Postural control

Sub-occipital Muscles located within the posterior aspect of the cervical spine in the sub- occipital region, right underneath the skull. Helps to maintain head position and head movement. See Table 1.3 for their function.

- Rectus capitis posterior (major and minor)
- Obliquus capitis (superior and inferior)

Table 1.3 Sub occipital Muscles

Muscle	Function
Rectus capitis posterior major	• Rotation of head to same side • Head extension
Rectus capitis posterior minor	• Head extension
Obliquus capitis inferior	• Head extension and flexion to same side
Obliquus capitis superior	• Head and neck rotation

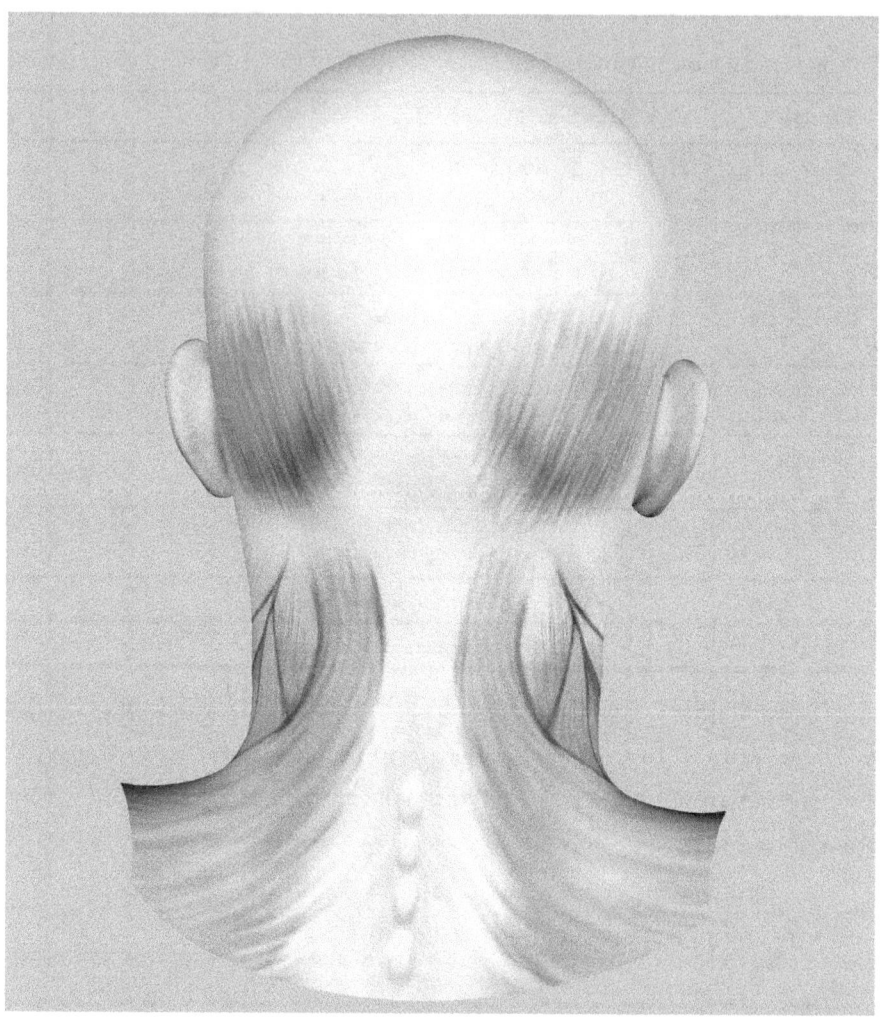

Sacrum and Coccyx Muscles are important in stabilizing the base of the spine. I will only mention the muscles that are originated from the spine, sacrum and/or coccyx. See Table 1.4 for their functions.

- Coccygeus
- Erector Spinae Muscles (Iliocostalis, Longissimus, and Spinalis)
- Gluteus Maximus
- Levator ani
- Multifidus

- Piriformis
- Psoas (minor and major)

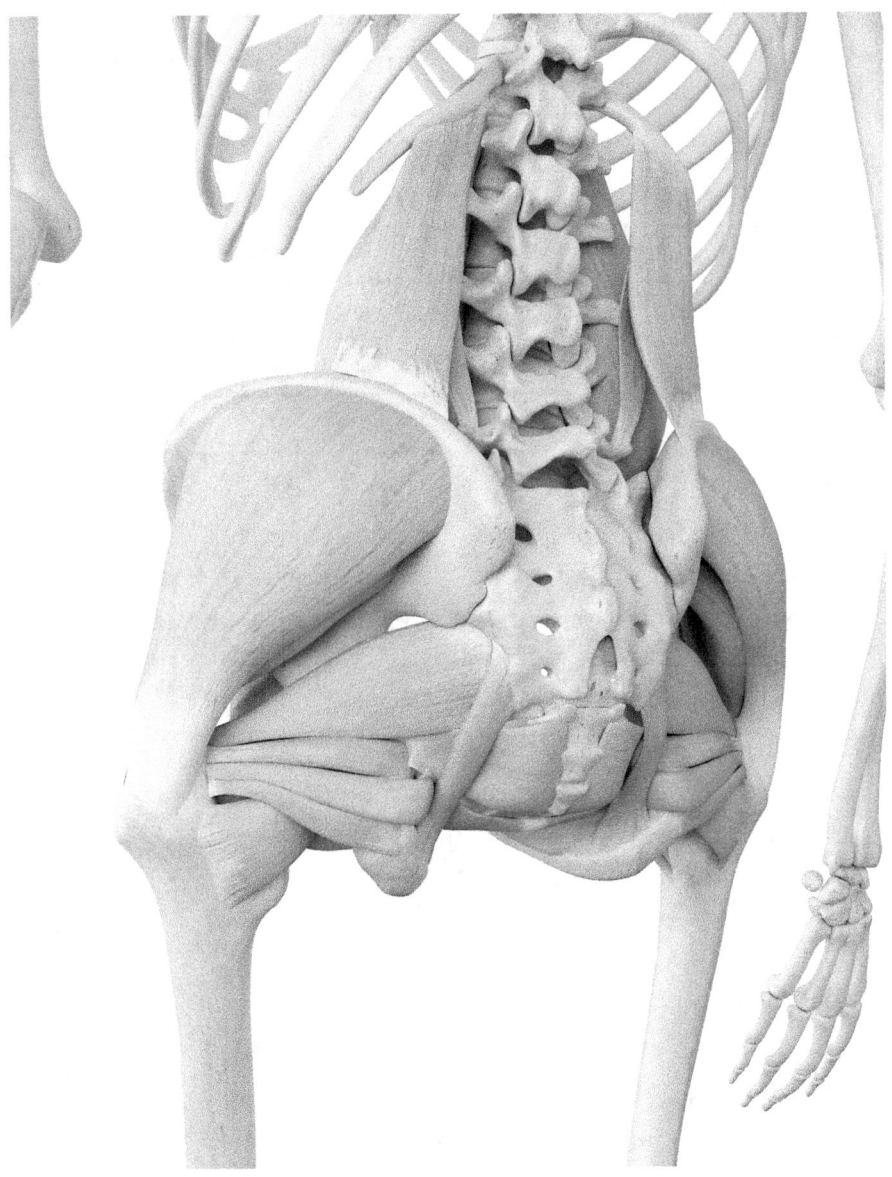

Table 1.4 Sacrum Muscles	
Muscle	Function
Coccygeus	• Movement of coccyx.
Erector Spinae	• Extends the vertebral column.
Glueus Maximus	• Extension and external hip rotation.
Levator ani	• Supports organs in the pelvic cavity.
Multifidus	• Stabilize the vertebral column.
Piriformis	• External rotation of the hip.
Psoas major	• Flex and laterally rotate hip.
Psoas minor	• Trunk flexion.

Skeletal muscles work by moving bones and they do so by pulling. A skeletal muscle can shorten, lengthen or stay the same. When a skeletal muscle contracts it shortens, decreasing the joint space between two bones pulling them closer together. When a skeletal muscle relaxes it lengthens. There are twenty muscle groups located in the posterior (back) of the body, from the back of the skull to the posterior pelvis. These muscles all play an important role in maintaining your posture as you move through different body positions. If one of these muscles are weakened as a result of an injury or become too tight/spastic because of over-stimulation they will alter your posture position.

You Should Know:
- Skeletal muscles maintain and move your body through different body positions.
- Muscles move bones into different positions by contracting.
- The deep intrinsic back muscles are commonly injured during improper lifting technique.
- You are more likely to injury yourself when your muscles become fatigued.

Chapter 2

What Causes Back Pain?

"The greatest evil is physical pain."

Saint Augustine

According to the National Institute of Health, eight out of ten people will experience back pain at some point in their lives. There are many factors that can cause back pain. To determine the exact cause of back pain, an examination is performed and additional testing (e.g. x-ray, MRI) may be required. Once the cause is determined the type of treatment recommended will be based on the cause. Back pain remains one of the leading causes of medical visits as well as the number one reason why people miss work. If you are experiencing back pain it doesn't have to be a lifetime issue if detected and treated early.

Understanding Pain

The definition of pain, according to Merriam-Webster Dictionary, pain is *"localized physical suffering associated with bodily disorder (as a disease or an injury); also: basic bodily sensation induced by a noxious stimulus, received by naked nerve endings, characterized by physical discomfort (as pricking, throbbing, or aching), and typically leading to evasive action."*

Pain is your perception. It's what is perceived by your brain at the moment; therefore, it is completely subjective. What may be perceived as painful to you can be perceived as enjoyable for another person. For this reason, there are different types of pain and different thresholds for pain. When a stimulus becomes overwhelming or too much it becomes painful. Pain is a term used to describe a response by the nervous system. You may feel sharp, dull, ache, or numbness and tingling. Depending on the description of your pain, it can help with determining the cause of your pain. For example, ache, stiff and dull pain can be muscle or joint related.

Poor Posture

Sit up straight! Don't slouch! are examples of phrases you've heard your parents say repeatedly while sitting at the dinner table. Not only is poor posture taxing to the body and it makes you appear older than what you really are, it tells what is going on with your muscles. Are you favoring one side because you have pain or discomfort?

Poor posture can be created by: weakened muscles, scoliosis, or spinal arthritis.

The Wrong Mattress

We spend the majority of our lives sleeping. Investing in a good mattress maybe just what you need to reduce your back pain. How would you describe your night? Are you restless? Do you spend most of your time tossing and turning? Is your body sore, achy or stiff in the morning? I know I sound like a mattress commercial, but sleeping is essential and getting sound sleep is very important.

It's not the quantity or the amount of hours you sleep but the quality. Are you going into the deep stages of sleep, REM? During this phase of sleeping your body is healing and repairing from a day of work. Your body releases growth hormone, which helps in the repairing process. When we do not get adequate sleep, we awaken with a stiff neck or back and some of us have to literally roll out of bed in the morning. That is no way to start your day... in pain. Do yourself a favor. Get rid of the old lumpy mattress. Maybe you need a soft mattress or maybe a firm one. Visit your local mattress store, try out a few and invest in a good mattress. Your back will love you for it.

Bone or Joint Disease

Conditions such as spinal arthritis can also cause back pain. However, I've seen cases were a patient have spinal arthritis and not experience any pain or discomfort. Located within the joints, muscles, soft tissue (ligaments, tendons), bones, skin and other joints are pain receptors called nociceptors. These receptors respond to extreme temperatures (hot/cold), mechanical (pressure, crushing), and chemical stimuli. When these receptors are damaged like in the case of disc disease, it can lead to pain being perceived by the person.

Muscle Strain (Acute or Chronic)

Overuse injury, improper use or trauma causes muscle strain. Muscles strain is the most common cause of back pain. You are more likely to injure yourself when you are fatigued. When your muscles become tired, it cannot support your body adequately as a result, they become overworked and over stretched and tear, leading to a strain. A muscle strain is a result of damage to the muscles, tendons or muscle fibers. Using improper lifting technique repetitively can cause back pain. Not only are you loading your back with excessive weight, but if you are tired or fatigued while attempting to lift fifty pounds from the floor, you can very easily damage your back.

Your Occupation
Prolong Standing and/or Walking

Jobs that require prolong standing and/or walking include waitress, teacher, bartender, and security guard. Spending a third of your day on your feet can cause acute back pain. While standing, your lower back muscles are in constant contraction to help you maintain an upright posture and will eventually become fatigued. Most of the time, you do not feel the back pain until you sit down.

Prolong Sitting

Jobs that require prolong sitting include bank teller, clerical, business administrative, truck driving, bus operator, etc. Compared to prolong standing and/or walking, prolong sitting is actually worse for you. Not only does it tighten your flexor muscles (such as hip flexors, hamstrings and pectoral muscles), recent research has shown that it decreases your quality of life. Most people whose jobs require prolong sitting experience headache, neck and upper back pain.

Repetitive Lifting, Bending, Pulling, or Twisting

Manual labor jobs such a warehouse or construction worker, requires repetitive lifting, bending, pulling and twisting. Putting your body into various positions while lifting a load can lead to injury. Although most companies are required to have job safety training, you cannot overlook the fact that more than 4.1 million workers suffer from job-related injuries every year.

In Phase III, I discuss how you can improve muscle strength and endurance, which will help to reduce your chances of back injury.

Pregnancy

Back pain in pregnancy is usually the result of gaining weight rapidly. Due to the fact that the woman is gaining weight at a fast pace, it does not allow her body time to adjust to the changes.

Overweight and Obesity

An estimated 35 percent of people living in the U.S. are considered either overweight or obese. Unlike during pregnancy, this type of weight gaining is done gradually over a period of time. In the beginning the person may not experience back pain, but as time progress pain appears. Carrying excessive abdominal weight takes a toll on the body. Not only does it rob you of your energy, but it also places stress on the internal organs. In addition, it puts you at a greater risk for health problems such as diabetes and cardiovascular disease. If you or someone you love is overweight or obese, act now and do something about it. Your life depends on it.

Poor Physical Fitness

Physical fitness is very important in maintaining a healthy lifestyle. Being active is essential to living an active life. If you are not physically fit, chances are you do not exercise on a regular basis. Poor physical fitness can lead to weak muscles. Weak muscles can cause poor posture and increase your likelihood of injury.

You Should Know:
- Many things cause back pain. Some of which can be prevented, like being overweight or obese.
- Your lifestyle and occupation can contribute to back pain.

Chapter 3
What to Do

When you are injured and don't know what to do... ask for help.

If you suffer from an injury to your back the first thing to do is stop doing whatever is creating the back pain. Continuing to do the thing that is causing the back pain will only lead to further damage. If your injury is a result of a motor vehicle accident, slip-and-fall, or job-related injury, seek help right away. In this case, because it is a physical trauma, the sooner you get help the better.

Normally back pain should go away after a week, however, if the pain has not changed or if the pain gets worse then you should seek the help of a licensed healthcare professional.

Home Care Instructions

I typically give home care instructions to patients to help them manage the pain in between appointments. For a muscle strain injury, RIC (Rest Ice Compression) is very effective and appropriate to do for the first forty-eight to seventy-two hours. The goal for the first seventy-two hours is to reduce swelling and prevent further damage. Moist heat can be utilized after seventy-two hours to help promote tissue healing by increasing blood flow to the area. The application of moist heat too soon can result in more pain. Although the heat may feel soothing and relaxing while it is being used, when removed the muscles tighten up creating more pain and discomfort.

Rest

Rest from any activity that would exacerbate or worsen the pain. Rest does not mean sitting on the sofa all day or lying in bed. Continue to do what you would normally do, just don't overdo it. Avoid strenuous and repetitive activities.

Benefits of Resting:
- Reduce the chances of making the injury worse.
- Allows proper healing to take place.

Ice

Using ice for the first forty-eight to seventy-two hours post-injury can be very beneficial. Apply ice to the area for ten to fifteen minutes, every hour to reduce swelling. Avoid using heat and analgesic creams during this time. After seventy-two hours, you can use heat packs to help promote blood flow to the area helping the healing process.

Benefits of Ice Therapy:
- Reduce swelling and inflammation.
- Causes muscles spasm which helps push fluid and edema away from the injured area.
- Numbs the area and may provide temporary pain relief.

Compression
Compression is used to decrease swelling and the accumulation of fluid

and edema within the injured area. It also helps stabilize the area to prevent further tissue damage, by not allowing you to move too freely.

Let Chiropractic Be Your First Choice

Oftentimes patients come into the office with chronic back pain who only sought our services because we were their last choice. After conducting a history on a patient I would discover that their pain started out as an annoying ache that they have been self-medicating for years. The pain would go away for a while and something would cause it to flare up, for an example shoveling snow or driving extensively. They would go on to say, that when the pain returned it felt like the first day the back pain began. They would take medication, the pain would go away and they would move on with their lives. The pain would flare up again after doing some form of activity and now they are back to square one. They begin this vicious cycle of episodic flare-ups for years, until finally the pain returns one day but the medication no longer works. The medicine is not working, now they do not know what to do.

The goal of chiropractic care is not only to get you out of pain as quickly as possible but to improve your overall function.

Chiropractic care is a safe, non-invasive approach to relieve musculoskeletal pain without the side-effects that are seen when taking medicine.

You Should Know:
- If your pain does not improve or change after one week, seek professional help.
- Consider the help of a licensed Chiropractor; we specialize in treating musculoskeletal injuries such as neck, back and joint pain.
- Rest, ice, and compress the injured area for the first seventy-two hours to reduce swelling.

Chapter 4
What You Should NOT Do

*"Remember that pain has this most excellent quality. If pro-
longed it cannot be severe, and if severe it cannot be prolonged."*

Seneca

As I stated before, don't continue to do the activity that created your
back pain. Remember, you want to decrease further damage to the injured area; therefore, taking it easy and following the *RIC* protocol for
the first seventy-two hours are essential.

Wait until the Pain is Worse
Don't wait until the pain becomes chronic (meaning you've had it for
more than three months) to seek help. Many people will self-medicate
and will only seek help when the pain has become debilitating. In order
to prevent an injury from becoming chronic you should consider seeking help immediately after an injury occurs. This will allow you to get
the proper guidance you need in order to have a speedy recovery.

Continue to Self-Medicate with No Results
Over the past ten years, there has been an increase in the dependency

of prescription pain medicine. If you are taking medicine and it is not working, then I recommend you to try something else. Continuing to do something that does not yield the results you want is pointless. With the vast amount of information available to you today, at the touch of a finger, you have alternative choices. Search your options and take action.

Special Note: Please consult with your medical doctor prior to discontinuing any prescribed medication.

Avoid Professional Help

"I don't like the doctor," "All they do is take my money, and do nothing." These are some of the excuses I've heard over the years, to justify why people don't seek help. Missing days from work, not being able to do the things you enjoy are good reasons why you should seek help sooner. Back pain is one of the leading causes of permanent disability in the United States. Seeking immediate help right after an injury has occurred rather than later can be the difference between returning to work and not returning to work.

You Should Know:
- Don't wait until the pain is debilitating. Seek help sooner.
- If the pain is getting worse or changing, the injury maybe more serious than you thought.
- If you are experiencing radiating pain, such as numbness, tingling or pins and needles seek help.
- Consult with your medical doctor prior to discontinuing any prescribed medication.

Chapter 5

The Difference between Acute and Chronic Pain

"Pain is such an uncomfortable feeling that even a tiny amount of it is enough to ruin every enjoyment."

Will Rogers

Acute Pain

Acute pain is a sudden onset of pain and usually sharp in nature, that will usually get you to stop doing whatever you were doing. It's a signal to you that something has gone wrong. One day a patient walked into the office, bent over with one hand on his lower back. Moving slowly, he shuffled his way to the seat and sat down. After he was directed into the examination room, he informs me that he was bending over to remove a boat battery and felt an intense sharp pain in his lower back. His exact words were, "It felt like I've been stabbed." He said he dropped the battery immediately and just stood stooped over for fifteen minutes because he could not move.

Acute back pain generally last from a couple of weeks to three months and is self-limiting. It is generally associated with skeletal muscle spasm, swelling, edema and soft tissue injury. If treated early, acute back pain may not progress to chronic back pain. If the back pain has not changed or is getting worse, seek the help of a licensed healthcare professional. Acute pain is usually not associated with an underlying disease, most of the time it is a result of recent trauma or injury. Examples of acute back pain would be a herniated disc or back pains during child labor.

Chronic Pain

Chronic pain is a gradual occurrence that may result in an underlying disease present. Back pain becomes chronic when you have recovered and the tissues have healed but you continue to experience pain. Chronic back pain can last anywhere from three months to years. Typically it is diagnosed after having pain (reoccurring or long-lasting) for more than 6 months. In the United States, an alarming 30 percent of its residents suffer from chronic pain.

Those who suffer from chronic pain are at times not taken seriously. They are written off as "fakers" or told that "it is all in their heads" or that "their injury was long ago, and they should no longer be in pain." As a result, those who suffer from chronic back pain are more likely to be depressed, stressed, and feel hopeless. Examples of chronic back pain are Failed Back Surgery Syndrome, Fibromyalgia and Scoliosis.

You Should Know:
- Pain is normal and should not be ignored. It lets you know something is not right.
- Acute back pain is usually self-limiting. Lasting anywhere from a few weeks to three months.
- Pain is considered chronic at three months or greater.
- Chronic pain can be managed; there is hope, even if you had the pain for years.

Phase II
Rebuilding and Recovery

"Scars are not injuries, Tanner Sack. A scar is a healing.
After injury, a scar is what makes you whole."

China Mie'ville, *The Scar*

Introduction to Phase II

Once an injury has occurred it is important to undergo some form of rehabilitative program that helps to restore and improve function. Self-medicating is really not the only answer. Yes, the medication does help to reduce pain, relax the muscles and allow you to make it through your day, but does it really get rid of what is causing the back pain? The answer is no. Medicine merely hides the symptoms it doesn't get to the root of the problem. Let me make it clear, medicine does have an important role to play in the world, and I am thankful for that. However, we also should be aware of the other options we have of treating illnesses and diseases.

This phase explains why it is important to be active while your injury heals. Now this doesn't mean you should run a marathon or bike for twenty miles, it does mean that you can maintain a level of physical fitness that would not exacerbate or interrupt the healing process.

Chapter 6

Give It Time

*"A man too busy to take care of his health is like a mechanic
too busy to take care of his tools."*

Spanish Proverb

Fast-Paced Lives, Expecting Fast Healing

Living in the age of technology we have grown accustomed to instant gratification. If we want to lose weight, we can simply take a diet pill. Fast food, high-speed Internet, and microwave dinners, no wonder the majority of the people don't want to wait or don't have the patience to wait.

Our lives have become too busy and hectic leaving little to no room for us to simply enjoy life. When was the last time you went on an errand without your cell phone? Or had lunch with a friend, and the conversation wasn't interrupted by a text message notification? With that being said, people just don't have the patience to allow their bodies to heal. If you are experiencing pain, discomfort or disease within your body; it may seem convenient to go to the local pharmacy and purchase over-the-counter (OTC) medication. Okay, you get instant relief in some instances, but over a long period of time, taking the pain medicine such as Tylenol and Advil can lead to conditions such as liver disease. Now you have a whole other issue to deal with, in addition to the back pain.

We have become accustomed to demanding anything we want. Whenever we want it, and the thing we demand becomes available to us. We think that our bodies will do the same in respect to healing immediately, on-demand. However, if there is tissue damage, it will take time to heal and repair those tissues. How long it takes depends on a number of factors:

- Your age
- Your occupation
- Your lifestyle
- Your health status
- Your level of physical fitness
- Your nutritional intake
- The type of injury

It Takes Time to Heal
Give it time. Yes, time. Be patient. It takes the body time to heal. However long it takes for you to heal, trust your body enough to do what it was designed to do. The body is self-maintaining, self-sustaining, and self-healing. The body does not need any help, just no interference. Saying that you are too busy to seek care for yourself, or that you're busy so, you can't afford to relax, or that you have a spouse, children and other obligations. I get that; we all have obligations, but how well can you commit to those obligations if you are not in your best health condition?

Take Care of Yourself First
We must first learn to take care of ourselves before we can take care of

others. It is called self-preservation. As the flight attendant would say, please secure your own oxygen mask before helping others. You can take care of yourself by doing the following:

- Get plenty of sleep/rest.
- Eat a variety of foods.
- Drink water daily.
- Learn the art of meditation and practice it.
- Exercise at least a total of five hours a week.
- Quit smoking.

You Should Know:
- Be patient and allow the body to do what it does naturally. Heal.
- You cannot rush the healing process only assist it.
- Your health should be your number one priority.
- Help yourself first, and then you are in a better position to assist someone else.

Chapter 7

How the Body Heals

"'Healing,' Papa would tell me, 'is not a science, but the intuitive art of wooing nature.'"

W. H. Auden

The body is simply fascinating. Our mere existence on this planet is marvelous. The food we eat, the water we drink, and the air we breathe. We are equipped with all of the essentials to, not only survive, but to maintain living. We sometimes take the life we live, the health we have, and the people who love us for granted. Unaware that our world can be altered and changed at any given moment.

The body begins to heal immediately. There are three stages of healing: inflammatory (acute), repair, and remodeling. During the Inflammatory (Acute) Stage there is an increase of blood flow to the area. The blood brings oxygen, nutrients and chemicals that are important for tissue repair. This is also the stage that scar tissue began to form. Scar tissue is adhesive tissue that is seen during an injury. The muscles surrounding the injured site tighten or become spastic to limit movement and prevent further damage. As a result, fluid and edema begin to accumulate within and around the joints. The skin maybe warm to the touch, due to the increase of blood flow to the injured area.

Next, the body starts to lay down new connective tissue, collagen and blood vessels to help repair the damaged tissues. This stage is the Repair Stage. Scar tissue is still present at this moment, but there is a decrease in the amount of swelling in the area. During this stage, you can begin light stretches to help place stress on the scar tissue. This is a very important step. If there is no stress placed on the adhesive scar tissue it can restrict the range of motion of the joints. Therefore by stretching the muscles it breaks up the scar tissue.

The last stage of healing is the Remodeling Stage, there is little to no swelling or inflammation within or surrounding the joints of the injured area. The scar tissue is replaced by normal connective tissue along the stressed lines and there is an increased in joint motion. At this point, the patient is actively involved in their treatment. They are able to do exercises, which will help to strengthen the weakened muscles and help stabilize the supportive structures.

Table 7.1: Stages of Healing			
	Inflammatory (Acute)	**Repair**	**Remodeling**
Time:	1-3 days post-injury	4 days to 6 weeks	3 weeks to 12 months +
What you can do?	• Rest, ice, and compression • Avoid strenuous activity • Avoid heavy lifting • Avoid any activity that will make the pain worse	• Active light stretching • Iso-metric exercises • Ice then moist heat (10 minutes of ice followed by 10 minutes of heat). Always end with heat.	• Moderate stretching • Dynamic stretching • Iso-metric exercises • Moist heat
What the health-care professional can do?	• Give patient home care instructions (RIC). • Therapeutic modalities (e.g. Interferential Current, Ultrasound) • Kinesiotaping	• Therapeutic modalities • Passive stretching • Light joint mobilization	• Joint mobilization • Soft Tissue Therapy
Type of Care	Passive Care	Active Care	Active Care

You Should Know:

- Use ice during the acute stage to reduce the amount of swelling and inflammation.
- Add light stretching after four days to help break up adhesions (scar tissue).
- Use moist heat to help relax the muscles and reduce muscles spasm.
- Joint mobilization helps break up scar tissue (adhesions) and improve range of motion.

Chapter 8
Don't Just Sit Around

"Lack of activity destroys the good condition of every human being, while movement and methodical physical exercises save it and preserve it."

Plato

Doing Nothing Can Be Worse

Sitting on the sofa watching television for hours will make your back pain worse. Doing so maybe a good idea after back surgery, but after an acute injury it can potentially delay recovery. After an injury you should relax. Take a break from activities that would make the pain worse, avoid heavy lifting and other strenuous activities that would exacerbate the pain. If you are able to continue to go to work do so. Your life doesn't have to change because you have an injury. I'm not saying you should ignore the pain and push through it, but listen to your body. You alone know what you are able to handle.

Go back and read Chapter 3, "What to Do," then jump ahead and read Chapter 11: Beginner Program has exercises you can do after you have suffered an injury.

Back Braces Can Help

In my office I generally do not recommend patients to rest completely from activity. Most people who come into the office are either in acute or chronic pain. I typically will not give patients back braces, unless they really, really need it. For example, if their job requires prolong standing, walking, lifting, pulling, etc., then I would generally recommend they wear it while at work and remove it once they are home. The reason is this. By wearing the back brace, it provides additional support to the back muscles. The muscles are restricted from moving therefore limiting the motion of the back. As a result, after wearing the brace for 8 hours of the day, when the person finally removes it, the back pain will appear worse. Due to the fact that the muscles where restricted from moving and the brace provided the support rather than the muscles. If a patient is issued a back brace in my office, I typically start them on rehabilitative exercises as well to help strengthen the weakened muscles. The stronger the muscles become, the less likely they are in need of the back brace.

Exercises Can Help

In Phase III, there are different exercise programs that can be performed during each phase of healing. Light stretching and isometric exercises are effective in breaking up scar tissue and improving motion especially during the acute and sub-acute phase.

You Should Know:
- Lying and sitting around the house doing nothing can make the pain worse.
- Continue to do what you would normally do, just take precaution.
- Avoid any activity that would make the pain worse.
- Listen to your body. You alone know what you are able to handle so don't push yourself too hard.

Chapter 9

Know Your Treatment Options

"Self-education is, I firmly believe, the only kind of education there is."

Isaac Asimov

Back pain can be successfully managed and treated by various methods. There are many options available to you. If you have tried something and it did not work, do something else.

Complementary Alternative Medicine (CAM)
These are medical services that are not part of the standard medical care. These include doctors of chiropractic (D.C.), naturopathic physicians (N.D.) acupuncturist and message therapy (M.T.). They do not utilize medication or its products as a form of treatment of illnesses and diseases. However, in this section I will only discuss the benefits of chiropractic care and message therapy.

Chiropractic care is a great non-invasive and non-surgical way to treat and manage neck and back pain. Chiropractic care is not limited to just the back, but can be very effective in treating other joint pain such as shoulder and hip pain.

Chiropractic care is a form of health care that emphasize the restoration and maintaining of an individual's health through the adjusting of the spinal column. When an injury occurs to the back, fluid and edema accumulates within the joints. The fluid and edema contains substances that irritates the soft tissue (muscles, ligaments, and tendons) and irritate the nerve (spinal nerves), which can be expressed as tight and spastic muscles.

The chiropractor has the ability to help improve the motion within the spinal column through the application of a spinal adjustment. The adjustment can be done manually or by using a chiropractic instrument. Both are a high velocity maneuver that is applied to the spine to increase motion. As motion is restored and is improved within the spinal column (back), the fluid and/or edema that was accumulated is removed or pumped out. By doing so, the nerves are less or no longer irritated, resulting in normal toned muscle(s) that function better.

In addition, chiropractors may use therapeutic modalities such as heat or ice therapy, therapeutic ultrasound, or electrical muscle stimulation to help relieve pain and reduce muscle spasm prior to the spinal adjustment.

Most insurance plans, such as Blue Cross Blue Shield, Aetna, Cigna, and Medicare, cover chiropractic care. Check with your current health insurance company for more information.

Table 9.1 Chiropractic Care	
Benefits of Chiropractic Care	Risks of Chiropractic Care
• Decrease muscle tightness/spasm. • Increase joint range of motion. • Pain relief. • Break up scar tissue (adhesions). • Improve posture. • Restore and maintain balance. • Improve function	• Headache • Fatigue • Pain in the area treated.

Massage Therapy

Soft tissue therapy, such as massage therapy, has great benefits with no life threatening side-effects. Massage involves the manipulation of the muscle and connective tissues using a variety of techniques. It is used to treat musculoskeletal conditions such as neck and back pain.

Some side-effects from chiropractic care and massage therapy may be muscle soreness or ache at the side being treated.

Table 9.2 Massage Therapy	
Benefits of Massage Therapy	**Risks of Massage Therapy**
• Decrease muscle tightness/spasm. • Promote tissue healing. • Promote relaxation. • Pain relief. • Break up scar tissue (adhesions). • Increase lymphatic flows. • Increase blood flow. • Promote better sleep. • Stress reduction. • Reduce blood pressure and heart rate. • Reduce anxiety and depression.	• Temporary pain or discomfort. • Bruising. • Swelling. • Sensitivity or allergy to massage oils/lotions.

Conventional Medicine

This is your standard medical care, which include medical doctors (M.D.), doctors of osteopathy (D.O.) and allied health professionals such as nurses and physical therapists (P.T.). This form of medical services utilizes medication and/or surgery as its form of treatment of illnesses and diseases.

Medication: Muscle Relaxants and Nonsteroidal anti-inflammatory drugs (NSAID) including Ibuprofen

Medicine does have its benefits, but we should also be aware of the side-effects before consuming such drugs. Unfortunately we live in a society that is constantly influenced by the media to take medication. So, the first time a person experiences back pain, they usually take Advil or Tylenol. Unlike the forms of treatment mentioned under the CAM section, medicine comes with side-effect that can result in damage to any of the important internal organs (e.g. liver disease, stomach ulcers) if abused, misused, or overused.

From what I have experienced while practicing, the majority of people do not like to take medicine. Some patients didn't like how the medicine made them feel or they didn't want to become dependent on medicine. Sadly, they felt that was their only option and eventually they would resort to taking the medicine because that's all they knew at that time. Medicine is not the end-all answer to every ache, pain or condition our body may encounter, but it does serve many purposes.

If the benefits outweigh the risk, the Federal Drug Administration (FDA), will approve and deem that drug to be safe for public use. All drugs have risk, as with everything in life, therefore, necessary precautions must be considered before consuming such products. Consult with your medical doctor and other health care professionals to ensure that the potential of a negative reaction is low. Only take medicine as prescribed by your medical doctor, doing otherwise can be potentially harmful.

Muscles Relaxants are generally prescribed for musculoskeletal conditions such as a neck and back pain. Remember, muscle relaxants just don't relax the muscles in your back, but all muscles, including your heart muscles. Some side-effects maybe drowsiness and general fatigue.

Table 9.3 Muscle Relaxants	
Benefits of Muscle Relaxants	Risks of Muscle Relaxants
• Pain relief. • Reduce muscle spasm/tightness.	• Drowsiness or dizziness. • Possible addiction or dependency. • Dry mouth. • Urinary retention.

NSAID are also used to alleviate musculoskeletal pain but it can also be used to lower fevers.

Table 9.4 NSAID (including Ibuprofen)	
Benefits of Ibuprofen	**Risks of Ibuprofen**
• Pain relief. • Reduce fever. • Anti-inflammatory (decrease swelling).	• Upset stomach. • Nausea, drowsiness or dizziness. • Vomiting. • Diarrhea or constipation.

Back Surgery

Back surgery is not the first option in treating back pain. It only becomes necessary when the spinal nerves are compromised and thereby affecting its normal function. Compression of the spinal nerve can be a result of a disc protrusion (bulging or herniated) or bone spur (as seen in Osteoarthritis). This can result in numbness and tingling into the extremities, muscles weakness or atrophy or the inability to control urinary/bowel function. In this case, back surgery may be deemed necessary. In addition, those individuals who may benefit from spinal surgery are those who have not responded to the reasonable effort to relieve pain, including medication and alternative medical treatment.

Otherwise, it is rarely necessary to have back surgery to relieve localized back pain. In some cases back surgery fails and the person continues to experience back pain, Failed Back Surgery Syndrome (FBSS).

Table 9.5 Back Surgery	
Benefits of Back Surgery	**Risks of Back Surgery**
• Relieves pain. • Reduce radicular pain.	• Feeling of numbness and tingling. • Continued pain. • Restricted or loss of range of motion or stiffness. • Spinal degeneration around surgical site. • Heart and lung complications (general surgery risk). • Excessive bleeding or infection (general surgery risk).

Spinal Injections

Local injections of anti-inflammatory steroids into the spinal area have been used to treat lower back pain. The amount of relief varies from person to person, and has its risk and benefits as well.

Table 9.6 Spinal Injections	
Benefits of Spinal Injections	**Risks of Spinal Injections**
• Relieves pain. • Improve function.	• Increased pain. • Headache. • Nerve injury (rare). • Infection (rare). • Bleeding (rare).

As you can see there are many treatment options available to help relieve your back pain; therefore do your research then decide what route to take. Take responsibility for your health, the health care professionals are only here to assist and guide you in the right direction.

You Should Know:

- Back pain can be treated and managed with different forms of healthcare.
- Educate yourself on the benefits and risk then make a choice.
- Healthcare professionals are here to serve you and support you in maintaining a level of optimal functional health by providing treatment, education and guidance. We do not heal you, that's your job.

Phase III

Preventing Back Pain with Exercise

"An ounce of prevention is worth a pound of cure."
Benjamin Franklin

Introduction to Phase III This phase will detail the exercises and stretches you should perform to prevent, eliminate and reduce neck and back pain. There are four exercise programs listed, that I have created that are beneficial to those patients who are under Passive (Relief) and Active (Conditioning) care.

During Passive (Relief) Care, in my office I use therapeutic modalities such as ice/moist heat, ultrasound, Kinesiotaping or interferential (muscle) stimulation, in conjunction with chiropractic adjustments. The goal at this time is provide pain relief. I generally give home care instructions to help the patient in-between doctors' visits. The patient may do light stretching. At this time, the doctor is doing most of the work; therefore, this is called Passive (Relief) Care.

After a period of time, which varies from patient to patient, once the patient's level of pain has decrease and they are showing signs of improvement, I move them into Active (Conditioning) Care. During this time, the patient is doing most of the work, they are now actively involved in their treatment and the doctor is doing less work. This is the time I usually institute active exercises and active stretching, based on the patients' level of tolerance.

The reason why patients are more prone to re-injury is because of weak muscles and inflexibility. The skeletal muscles have many functions, such as moving bones and maintaining posture and support to the joints. If there is a weakness in any of the back muscles, they are not able to do their jobs fully. If muscles are weak, it will become fatigue quickly and fail. The failure of the back muscles may not be noticed until you attempt to pick up a heavy object and you hear a "pop" in your back and you can't stand up straight. How miserable is that? Who wants to experience that? Not me, and I'm sure you don't either. The key to preventing this type of scenario from happening to you is a rehabilitation program that includes strength training and flexibility exercises.

Flexibility is important in maintaining range of motion within the joints. The more flexible you are, the muscles, tendons and ligaments can go a great length before they are stressed or overstretched.

This phase will equip you with the necessary exercises and stretches you can perform at home to manage back pain. The exercises are for the entire back, including, the neck, mid-back, lower back and sacrum regions.

Chapter 10
Beginner Program

"I like exercise. I like a healthy body."

Erin Gray

Here are some great beginner exercises and stretches you can do to get you started to conditioning your muscles. Whether you have just suffered from an injury or you're having a flare-up, this is a great place to begin. Ideally, you should warm-up prior to doing any of the exercise programs. Walk in place for five to ten minutes and control your breathing. It's a very light, easy walk, so no panting. Once you feel your body is warm and ready, begin exercising.

Beginner Program for the Cervical Spine (Neck)
These exercises can be performed standing or seated. Always begin each exercise in the neutral position with your head and eyes facing forward.

Dynamic Cervical Stretches

Ear-to-Shoulder: Start in a neutral position. Slowly bend your head to the right, bringing your ear to your shoulder then to the left, alternating from side to side. Do three sets of ten to fifteen repetitions.

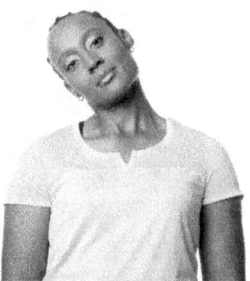

Head Rotation: Start in a neutral position. Slowly turn your head to the right, as if looking over your shoulder, then to the left, alternating from side to side. Do three sets of ten to fifteen repetitions.

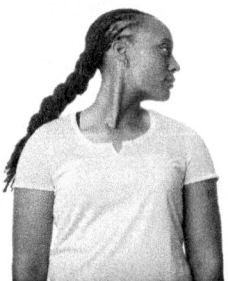

Head Nod: start in a neutral position. Slowly bring your head back (as if you're trying to touch your back with the back of your head) then lower your head forward bringing your chin to your chest without tucking your chin. Do three sets of ten to fifteen repetitions.

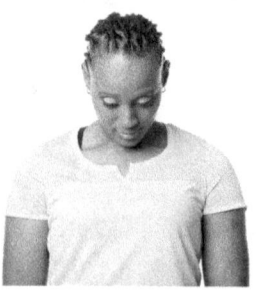

Static Cervical Stretches

Four-Point Stretch: start in a neutral position.

- Point 1: Drop your head forward bringing your chin to your chest, now place both hands behind your head pushing downward until you feel the stretch. Hold for thirty count. Take a deep breath in, as you exhale push down further and hold for thirty count, then release. Repeat three times.

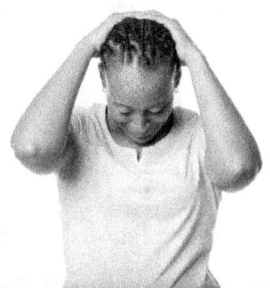

- Point 2: Point your head downward toward your right leg, now place your right hand on the left side of your head until you feel the stretch. Hold for thirty count. Take a deep breath in, as you exhale, push down further and hold for thirty count, then release. Repeat on the left side. Repeat three times.

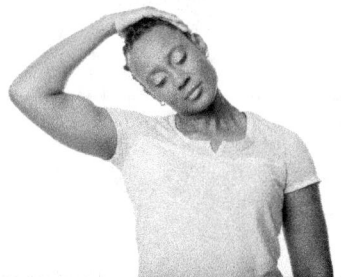

- Point 3: Bend your head to the right, bringing your right ear towards your right shoulder, now place your right hand on the left side of your head until you feel the stretch. Hold for thirty count. Take a deep breath in, as you exhale, push down further and hold for thirty count, then release. Repeat on the left side. Repeat three times.

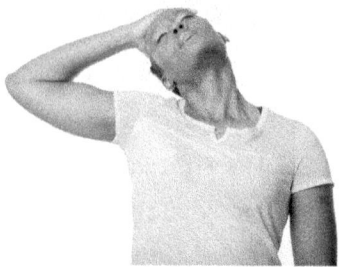

- Point 4: Bend your head backward, as if you were touching your back with the back of your head. With your hands in a prayer position, place your fingertips at the bottom of your chin and push upward until you feel the stretch. Hold for a thirty count. Take a deep breath in, as you exhale, push up further and hold for a thirty count, then release. Repeat three times.

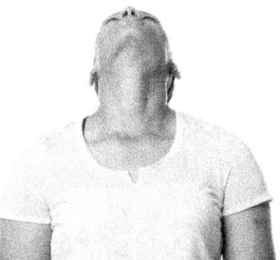

Cervical Exercises
Cervical Extensions: Start in a neutral position. Interlock your fingers then place them behind your head. Extend your head backwards, as if you are looking up to the ceiling. Do three sets of ten to fifteen repetitions.

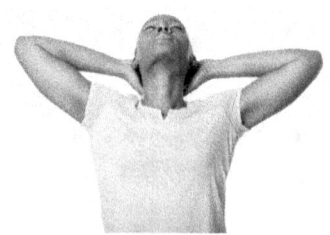

Neck Push-1: Start in a neutral position. Interlock your fingers then place them behind your head (in the center). Push your head against the resistance of your hands for ten count hold, then release. Repeat for a total of ten times.

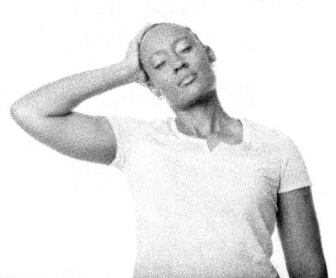

Neck Push-2: Start in a neutral position (head and eyes facing forward). Take your right palm and place it on the side of your head (above the ear). Push your head to right against the resistance of your hand and hold for ten count, then release. Repeat for a total of ten times on this side then repeat on the left side.

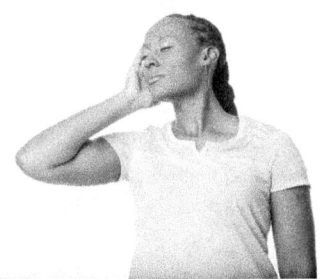

Beginner Program for the Thoracic Spine (Mid-Back)
These exercises can be performed standing or seated. Always begin each exercise in the neutral position with your head and eyes facing forward.

Static Thoracic Stretches

Hug: Stretch your arms out by your side then bring them in, giving yourself a big hug. Hold for thirty count then release. Repeat five times.

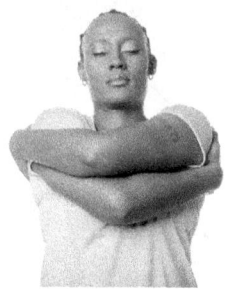

Hug-and-Tuck: Give yourself a hug, tuck your chin towards your chest then bend forward at the waist. Hold for thirty count then release. Repeat for five times.

Thoracic Exercises Shoulder Shrugs: Shrug your shoulders upward (bringing your shoulders toward your ears). Do three sets of ten to fifteen repetitions.

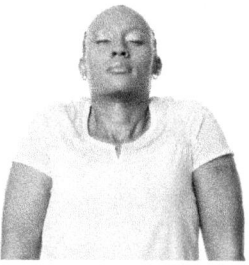

Shrug-and-Hold: Shrug your shoulders upward and hold for a ten count, then release. Repeat for ten times.

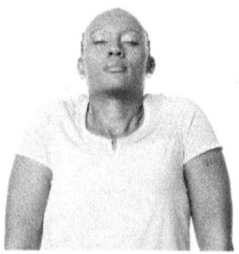

Shoulder Blade Squeeze: With your elbows bent, squeeze your shoulder blades together (as if you are trying to touch your elbows). Hold for ten count, then relax. Repeat ten times.

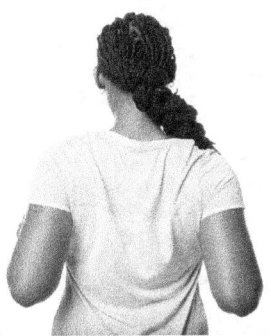

Peacock: In a seated position, sit on the edge of the seat. Start in a slouched position then slowly lifting your chest upward until you are sitting up straight. Hold in this position for ten count, then relax. Repeat for ten times.

Table 10.2 Beginner Program for the Thoracic Spine (Mid-back)	
Thoracic Stretches	**Thoracic Exercises**
• Hug • Hug-and-Tuck	• Shoulder Shrugs • Shrug-and-Hold • Shoulder Blade Squeeze • Peacock

Beginner Program for the Lumbar Spine (Low Back)

These exercises should be performed on the floor. Always begin each exercise in the neutral position lying on your back. Perform both the lumbar exercises and the sacrum exercises for maximum benefit.

Static Lumbar Stretches Knee-to-Chest 1: Bend your knees placing your feet on the floor. Place your right hand behind your right thigh, slowly bring your knee towards your chest until you feel the stretch.

Hold for thirty count, release then do the same on the left side. Repeat for five times.

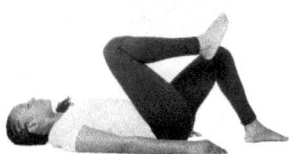

Knee-to-Chest 2: Bend your knees placing your feet on the floor. Placing both hands behind your thighs, slowly bring your knees toward your chest until you feel the stretch in the lower back. Hold for thirty count, then release. Repeat for five times.

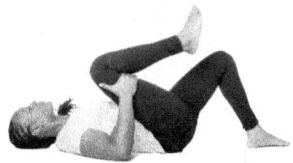

Dynamic Lumbar Stretches Knee-to-Chest 3: Bend your knees placing your feet on the floor. Alternate by bring your right and left knee towards your chest, one knee at a time as if you were marching. Keeping your knees bent. Do not straighten your leg. Do three sets of ten to fifteen repetitions.

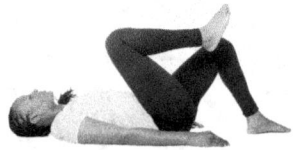

Lumbar Exercises

Abdominal Hallowing: Bend your knees placing your feet on the floor. Take a deep breathe in, allowing your belly to fill with air. As you exhale, push the air out while tightening your abdominal muscles, pushing your lower back into the floor. Hold for a count of ten, then relax. Do three sets of ten to fifteen repetitions.

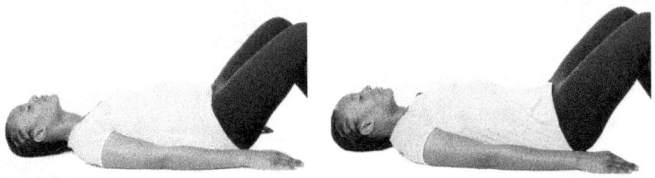

Pelvic Lift: Bend your knees placing your feet on the floor. Placing your hands by your side, palms down. Now, lift your hips upward towards the ceiling, go as high as you can, squeezing your glute muscles (buttocks) at the top, and then lower your hips back to the floor. That is one repetition. Do three sets of ten to fifteen repetitions.

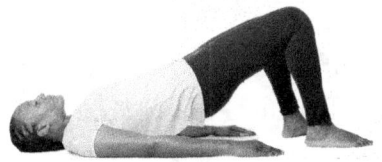

Table 10.3 Beginner Program for the Lumbar Spine (Lower Back)	
Lumbar Stretches	Lumbar Exercises
Static Stretches • Knee-to-Chest 1 • Knee-to-Chest 2 *Dynamic Stretches* • Knee-to-Chest 3	• Abdominal Hallowing • Pelvic Lift

Beginner Program for the Sacrum and Pelvis

These exercises should be performed on the floor. Always begin each exercise in the neutral position lying on your back, unless otherwise indicated. A physio ball will be needed.

Sacrum and Pelvis Static Stretch Piriformis Stretch: This stretch can be performed in a seated or lying position. Bend and grab your right knee bringing it across your body until you feel a stretch in the buttock region. Hold for thirty count, release. Repeat five times. Then do the left side.

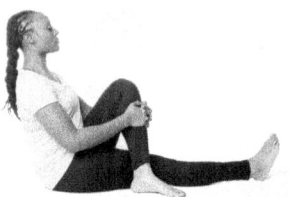

Hamstrings Stretch: This stretch can be performed seated, standing or lying on your back. Straighten the right leg, bend forward at the waist (avoid rounding your back) and bring your chest toward the direction of your toe. You should feel a stretch in the back of your thigh and lower leg (calf). Hold for thirty count, release. Repeat five times. Then do the left side. For a better stretch, use a towel or stretching strap.

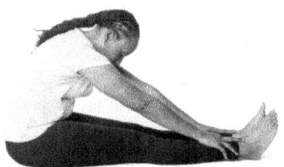

Quadriceps Stretch: This stretch can be performed lying on your side or standing. Bend the right knee, holding at the foot pull the foot in an upward motion. You should feel a stretch in the front of your thigh. Hold for thirty count. Repeat five times, then do the left side.

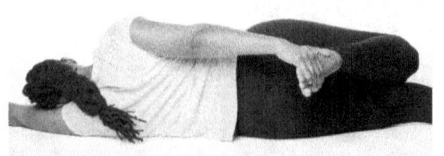

Sacrum and Pelvis Exercises

Pelvic Rock-N-Roll with Physio Ball: Sit on the ball with your feet shoulder width apart. Once you are balanced, move only your hips and pelvis and keep your upper body still. Perform the following exercises performing three sets of ten to fifteen repetitions for each one:

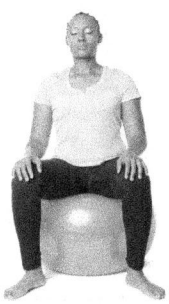

A. Side Rock: Rock your hips from side to side.

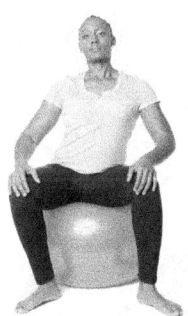 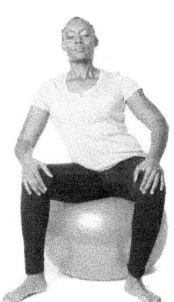

B. Swoops: Rock your hips back and forward. Do three sets of ten to fifteen repetitions

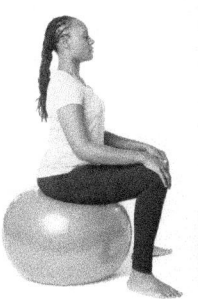 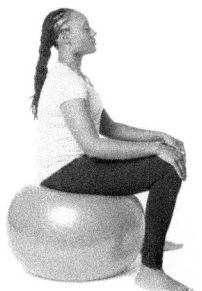

C. Clockwise Circles: Swirl your hips around in a clockwise motion.

D. Counter-Clockwise Circles: Swirl your hips around in a counter-clockwise motion, just like during exercise C.

Table 10.4 Beginner Program for the Sacrum and Pelvis	
Sacrum and Pelvis Stretches	**Sacrum and Pelvis Exercises**
• Piriformis Stretch • Hamstrings Stretch • Quadriceps Stretch	• Pelvic Rock-N-Roll with Physio Ball —Side Rock —Swoops —Clockwise Circles —Counter-Clockwise Circles

Once you are able to perform these exercises with little to no effort, move on to the next program, Intermediate Program. You can also make it more challenging by increasing the amount of repetitions for each exercise.

You Should Know:

- The Beginner Program is great for those individuals who are in acute pain or who are experiencing a flare-up (exacerbation).
- Take it easy and don't overdo it. Listen to your body and do what you can tolerate.
- Move on to the next program (Intermediate Program) when this program becomes easy to perform.
- You can make it challenging by increase the number of repetitions.

Chapter 11

Intermediate Program

"Start by doing what is necessary, then do what's possible, and suddenly you're doing the impossible."

Saint Francis of Assisi

Once the Beginner Program has become easier to do and it is no longer challenging to you, progress to the Intermediate Program. This program is designed for those individuals who are feeling at least 30-50 percent better or who suffer from chronic neck or back pain. Do what you can tolerate and listen to your body. Make sure that you warm up prior to doing any exercises like walking in place for five to ten minutes and control your breathing.

Intermediate Program for the Cervical Spine (Neck)
These exercises can be performed standing or seated. Always begin each exercise in the neutral position with your head and eyes facing forward. You will need resistance bands and/or small resistance ball. To maximize your efforts, first do the exercises from the Beginner Program then the exercises mentioned here.

Cervical Stretches: perform the same stretches from the Beginner Program.

Cervical Exercises Cervical Extension with Resistance Bands:
Placing the resistance band around the back of your head (centered).
Extend your head backwards, as if looking up to the ceiling. Do three
sets of ten to fifteen repetitions.

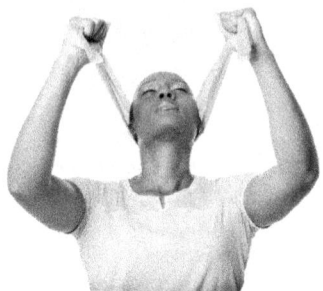

Cervical Extension with Physio Ball: Placing the ball in the back of
your neck. Extend your head backwards, pushing against the ball, as if
looking up to the ceiling. Do three sets of ten to fifteen repetitions.

Lateral Flexion with Resistance Bands: Placing the resistance band
around the right side of your head, positioned above the ear. Bend your
head to the right, bringing your ear towards your shoulder. Do three
sets of ten to fifteen repetitions. Repeat on the opposition side.

Lateral Flexion with Physio Ball: Place the ball on the right side of
your head above the ear. Bend your head to the right, pushing against
the ball. Do three sets of ten to fifteen repetitions. Repeat on the opposite side.

Forward Flexion with Physio Ball: Place the ball in the center of your
forehead. Bend your head forward, pushing against the ball. Do three
sets of ten to fifteen repetitions.

Table 11.1 Intermediate Program for the Cervical Spine (Neck)	
Cervical Stretches	Cervical Exercises
• See Beginner Program for the Cervical Spine	• Cervical Extension with Resistance Bands. • Cervical Extension with Physio Ball • Lateral Flexion with Resistance Bands • Lateral Flexion with Physio Ball • Forward Flexion with Physio Ball

Intermediate Program for the Thoracic Spine (Mid-Back)

These exercises can be performed lying face down, unless otherwise in-dicated. To maximize your efforts, first do the exercises from the Be-ginner Program then the exercises mentioned here.

Thoracic Stretches: perform the same stretches from the Beginner Program.

Thoracic Exercises

The Crow: Lying face down, extend your arms outward at a 90-degree angle. Now, lift both hands and arms off the floor at the same time. Do three sets of ten to fifteen repetitions.

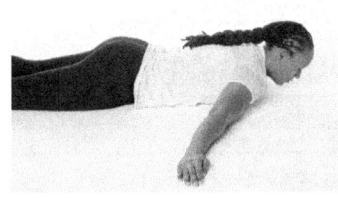 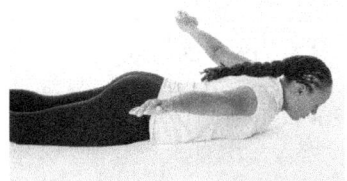

Rear Hand Clap: Lying face down, extend your arms outward at a 90-degree angle. Now, bring your hands together, as if clapping them be-hind your back. Do three sets of ten to fifteen repetitions. An alternative to this start with your arms by your side, then bring together, as if clapping your hands behind your back. Note: if you have shoulder problems or experience moderate pain or discomfort in the shoulders, avoid this exercise if it creates pain or discomfort.

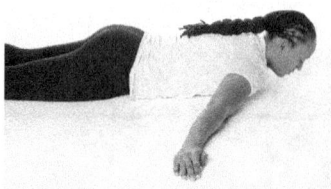 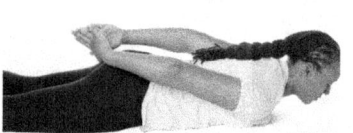

Scapular Retraction with Resistance Bands: Seated or standing with your arms out straight in front of you hold the resistance bands, open up your arms as if you are going to give someone a hug. Do three sets of ten to fifteen repetitions. Note: make sure you keep your arms at the height of your shoulders (90-degree angle).

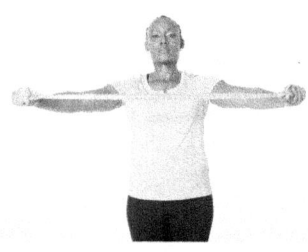

Table 11.2 Intermediate Program for the Thoracic Spine (Mid-Back)	
Thoracic Stretches	**Thoracic Exercises**
• See Beginner Program for the Thoracic Spine	• The Crow • Rear Hand Clap • Scapular Retraction with Resistance Bands

Intermediate Program for the Lumbar Spine (Lower Back)

These exercises can be performed while lying on your back in a neutral position, unless otherwise indicated. To maximize your efforts, first do the exercises from the Beginner Program then the exercises here. In addition, the Intermediate Program will include abdominal exercises that are helpful in stabilizing and strengthening the lower back.

Lumbar Stretches: perform the same stretches from the Beginner Program in addition to the stretches mentioned here.

Lumbar Twist: Bend your knees, crossing the right leg over the left. Allow your legs to fall to the left, bringing your knees to the floor. Hold for thirty count, then do the opposite side, crossing the left leg over the right, allow your legs to fall to the right. Repeat five times on each side.

Prayer Stretch: Kneeling on the floor. Extend your arms upward then bend forward at the waist. Hold for thirty count. Staying in this position, take a deep breath, try to go deeper into the stretch by bringing your buttocks toward your heels and walking your fingertips forward. Hold for thirty count. Repeat five times.

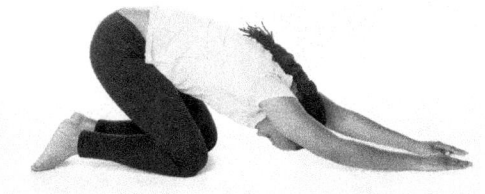

Cat Stretch: On your hands and knees. Taking a deep breath, drop your belly toward the floor extending your head backward. Now, exhale slowly while arching your back and tucking your chin towards your chest. Repeat five times.

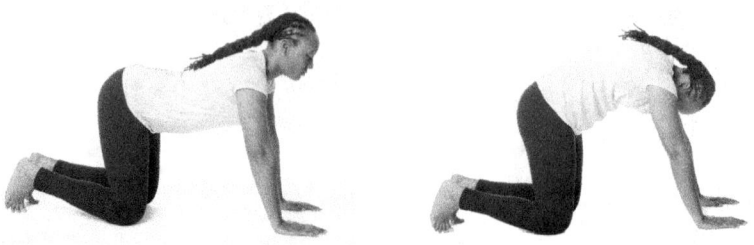

Lumbar Exercises

Knee-to-Chest 4: Lift your bent knee towards your chest. Alternating one leg at a time. Do three sets of ten to fifteen repetitions.

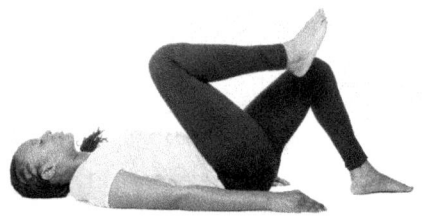

One-Leg Pelvic Lift: Lying on your back with your knees bent and feet flat on the floor. Extend your left leg. Now, lift your hips upward toward the ceiling. Repeat on the opposite leg. Do three sets of ten to fifteen repetitions.

Lumbar Twist with Physio Ball: Lying on your back with your knees bent, place the ball under your thighs. Place your arms by your side for stability. Squeezing the ball with your legs rotate the ball to the left going as far as you can without your shoulders rising off the floor. Then go to the opposition side, then back to the center. Do three sets of ten to fifteen repetitions.

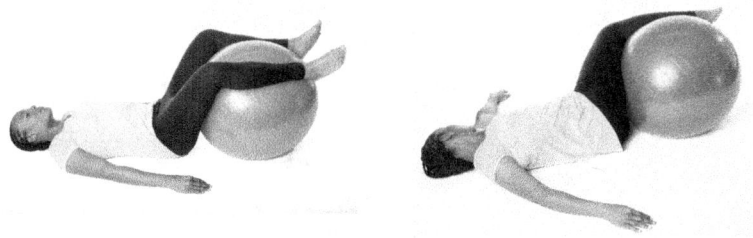

Back Extension: Lying face down with both arms by your side. Lift your head and upper body upward. Do three sets of ten to fifteen repetitions. Note: if your legs come off the floor while doing this, you may need to stretch your hamstrings.

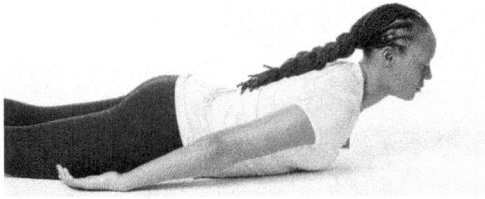

Modified Leg Lifts: Lying face down on the floor with both arms over your head and bend your knees. Lifting your leg (from the hip) toward the ceiling one leg at a time. Do three sets of ten to fifteen repetitions on each side.

Leg Lifts: Lying face down on the floor with both arms over your head and your legs straight. Lift your leg (from the hip) toward the ceiling one leg at a time. Do three sets of ten to fifteen repetitions on each side.

Abdominal Crunches: Lying on your back with your knees bent, place your hands on your thighs. Lift your chest toward your thighs. Do three sets of ten to fifteen repetitions. Note: Do NOT tuck your chin. Stick your chin outward when you make the crunch. Inhale in the start position and exhale in the end position.

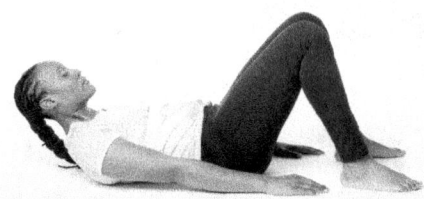

Modified Low Plank: Lying face down on the floor with your elbows bent and palms down by your side. Lift your body off the floor putting the weight onto your elbows and knees. Hold in this position thirty count. Relax and repeat five times. Note: Avoid sagging or hiking your hips. Your torso should be parallel to the floor. Remember to breathe. DON'T hold your breath!

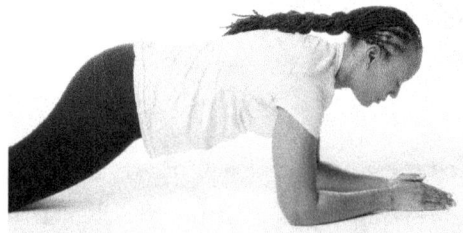

Low Plank: Lying face down on the floor with your elbows bent and palms down by your side. Lift your body off the floor putting the weight onto your elbows and balls of your feet. Hold in this position for thirty to sixty count. Relax and repeat three times. Note: Avoid sagging or hiking your hips. Your torso should be parallel to the floor. Remember to breathe. DON'T hold your breath!

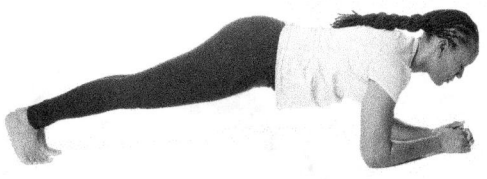

Table 11.3 Intermediate Program for the Lumbar Spine (Lower Back)	
Lumbar Stretches	**Lumbar Exercises**
• See Beginner Program for the Lumbar Spine • Lumbar Twist • Prayer Stretch • Cat Stretch	• Knee-to-Chest 4 • One-Leg Pelvic Lift • Lumbar Twist with Physio Ball • Back Extension • Modified Leg Lifts • Leg Lifts • Abdominal Crunches • Modified Low Plank • Low Plank

Intermediate Program for the Sacrum and Pelvis

Sacrum and Pelvis Stretches: Perform the same stretches from the Beginner Program.

Modified Side-Lying Leg Lifts: Lying on your left side with your knees bent. Extending from the hip, lift your right leg upward toward the ceiling. Repeat on the left leg. Do three sets of ten to fifteen repetitions.

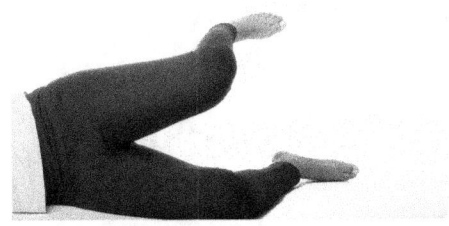

Side-Lying Leg Lifts: Lying on your left side with your legs straight. Lifting your leg (from the hip) toward the ceiling. Do three sets of ten to fifteen repetitions on each side.

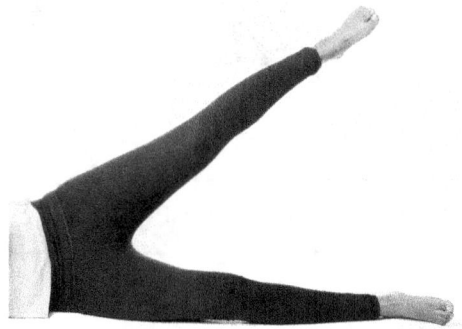

Modified Leg Lifts: Lying face down on the floor with both arms over your head and bend your knees. Lifting your leg (from the hip) toward the ceiling one leg at a time. Do three sets of ten to fifteen repetitions on each side.

Leg Lifts: Lying face down on the floor with both arms over your head and your legs straight. Lift your leg (from the hip) toward the ceiling one leg at a time. Do three sets of ten to fifteen repetitions on each side.

Ball Squeeze: Lying on your back with your knees bent and feet flat on the floor. Place the body ball between your knees. Now, squeeze both knees. Do three sets of ten to fifteen repetitions.

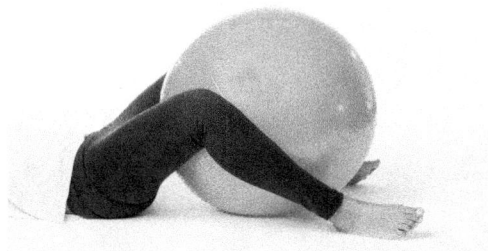

You Should Know:
- To get better results, combine the Beginner and Intermediate Programs.
- If the exercise becomes easy, increase the amount of repetitions or increase the time to make it more challenging.
- Move on to the Advanced Program, once you can do all the exercises in the Beginner and Intermediate Program with ease.
- Do the modified version if you have difficulty performing particular exercises (e.g. Modified Leg Lifts instead of Leg Lifts).

Chapter 12
Advanced Program

"Exercise doesn't get in the way of my life...it adds to the quality of it."

Unknown

This program is designed for those individuals who are 80 percent to 100 percent better. In addition, these exercises help to improve your balance and coordination. The exercises will help improve your strength as well as endurance. If you desire to increase your muscle mass then check out our Elite Program. Equipment needed: dumbbells and physio ball or wobble board. Make sure that you warm up prior to doing any exercises. Walk in place for five to ten minutes and control your breathing.

Advanced Program for the Cervical Spine (Neck)

Cervical Stretches: perform the same stretches from the Beginner and Intermediate Programs, in addition to the stretches mentioned here.

Star Gaze: Seated in a chair, allow your head to drop backward. Hold in this position for one minute. (Use a timer.) Keep adding time, until you build up to five minutes. Note: Adding time should be done progressively. For example, the first week, aim for one minute, the following add an additional minute and so forth.

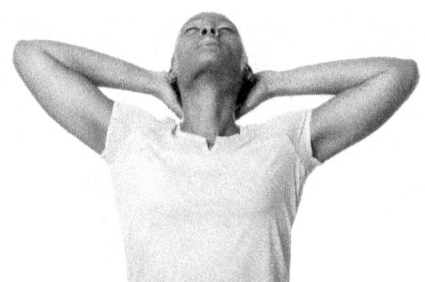

Cervical Exercises Cervical Extension (against gravity): Kneel over a chair or physio ball. Allow your head to drop forward, bringing your chin to your chest. Then extend your head backward. Do three sets of fifteen to twenty repetitions.

Table 12.1 Advanced Program for the Cervical Spine (Neck)	
Cervical Spine Stretches	Cervical Spine Exercises
• See Beginner Program for the Cervical Spine • Star Gaze	• Cervical Extension (against gravity)

Advanced Program for the Thoracic Spine (Mid-Back)

Thoracic Stretches: perform the same stretches from the Beginner and Intermediate Program.

Thoracic Exercises

The Crow with Dumbbells (on Physio Ball): Balance yourself facing down on the ball. With a dumbbell in each hand on the floor extended to the side. Lift your arms up. Do three sets of ten to fifteen repetitions.

Scapular Retraction with Dumbbells (on Physio Ball): Balance yourself facing down on the ball. With your arms bent at a 90-degree angle, lift the dumbbells off the floor. Keeping your elbows close to your body, squeeze your shoulder blades together. Do three sets of ten to fifteen repetitions.

Shoulder Shrugs with Dumbbells: This can be done in a seated, standing or on the physio ball or wobble board. Place dumbbell in each hand and relaxing your shoulders. Lift your shoulders upward towards your ears. Do three sets of ten to fifteen repetitions. Note: Do NOT move your head. Keep your head still during the exercises.

Table 12.2 Advanced Program for the Thoracic Spine (Mid-Back)	
Thoracic Spine Stretches	Thoracic Spine Exercises
• See Beginner Program for the Thoracic Spine	• The Crow w/ Dumbbells (on Physio Ball) • Scapular Retraction with Dumbbells (on Physio Ball or wobble board • Shoulder Shrugs with Dumbbells (seated, standing or on Physio Ball or wobble board)

Advanced Program for the Lumbar Spine (Lower Back)

Lumbar Stretches: perform the same stretches from the Beginner and Intermediate Programs.

Lumbar Exercises
Abdominal Crunches on Physio Ball: Sit on the ball now walk your feet forward while leaning your torso back until only your lower back is on the ball. Cross your arms over your chest now perform a crunch

bringing your elbows toward your knees. Do three sets of twenty to thirty repetitions.

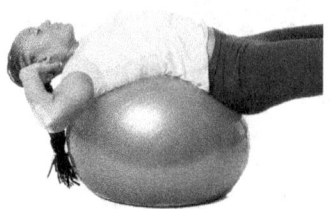 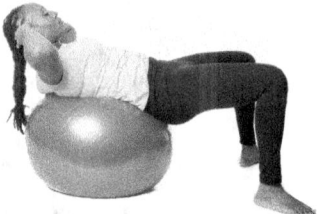

Back Extensions on Physio Ball: Place the ball underneath the front of your pelvis and balance yourself. Placing your arms by your side, balance the ball with your feet; now lift your chest off the ball. Do three sets of fifteen to twenty repetitions.

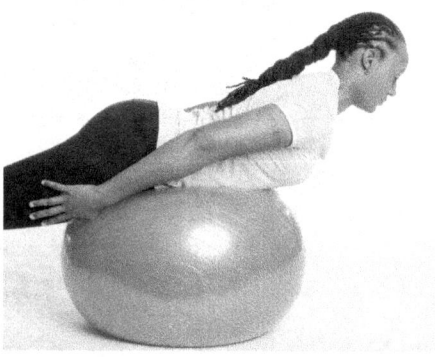

High Plank: Lying face down on the floor place your hands by your side with your elbows close to your body. Tuck your toes lifting your body off the floor, putting your weight onto your hands and balls of your feet. Hold for thirty to sixty count. Repeat three times. Note: Avoid sagging or hiking your hips. Your torso should be parallel to the floor. Remember to breathe. DON'T hold your breath.

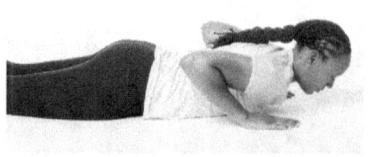 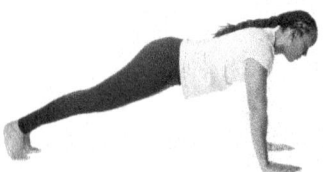

Low Plank on Physio Ball: Place both hands onto the ball with your elbows close to your body. Tuck your toes lifting your body off the ball, putting your weight onto your hands and the balls of your feet. Hold for thirty to sixty count. Repeat three times. Note: Avoid sagging or hiking your hips. Your torso should be parallel to the floor. Remember to breathe. DON'T hold your breath.

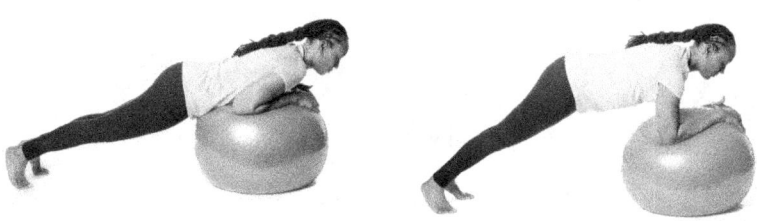

Pelvic Lift with Physio Ball: Lying face down on the floor with your legs straight. Place the ball under your feet/ankle. Now lift your hips upward toward the ceiling (end position). Do three sets of ten to fifteen repetitions.

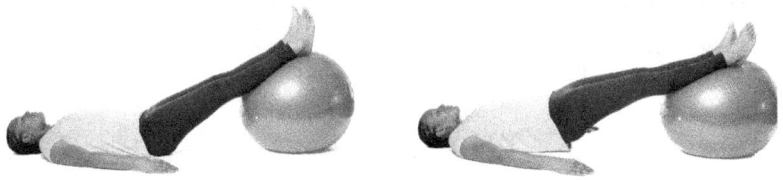

Low Plank Elbow-Knee Touch: Start in the Low Plank position. Alternate bringing your knee to your elbow on the same side (e.g. bring your right knee towards your right elbow). Do three sets of ten to fifteen repetitions.

High Plank Elbow-Knee Touch: Start in the High Plank position. Alternate bringing your knee to your elbow on the same side (e.g. bring your right knee towards your right elbow). Do three sets of ten to fifteen repetitions.

High Plank Elbow-Knee Touch (Opposite): Start in the High Plank position. Alternate bringing your opposite knee to the opposite elbow (e.g. bring your right knee towards your left elbow). Do three sets of ten to fifteen repetitions.

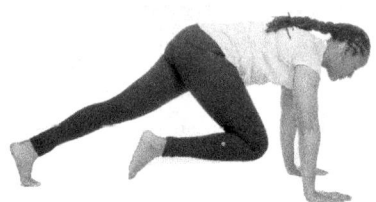

Advanced Program for the Sacrum and Pelvis
Sacrum and Pelvis Stretches: perform the same stretches from the Beginner and Intermediate Sacrum and Pelvis Programs.

Table 12.3 Advanced Program for the Lumbar Spine (Low Back)	
Lumbar Stretches	Lumbar Exercises
• See Beginner and Intermediate Programs for the Lumbar Spine	• Abdominal Crunches on Physio Ball • Back Extensions on Physio Ball • High Plank • Low Plank on Physio Ball • Pelvic Lift with Physio Ball • Low Plank Elbow-Knee Touch • High Plank Elbow-Knee Touch (Opposite)

Sacrum and Pelvis Exercises
Squats with Physio Ball: Position the ball between a wall and your lower back. Spread your feet shoulder width apart, now squat down. Do three sets of ten to fifteen repetitions. Note: Position your feet so that when you squat down, your knee does not pass your toes. If so,

readjust your position. AVOID leaning forward. Squat down as if you were sitting in a chair.

Sumo Squats (with or without Physio Ball): Start in the Squat position but this time spread your feet as wide as possible then squat down. Do three sets of ten to fifteen repetitions. Can be performed with or without the physio ball.

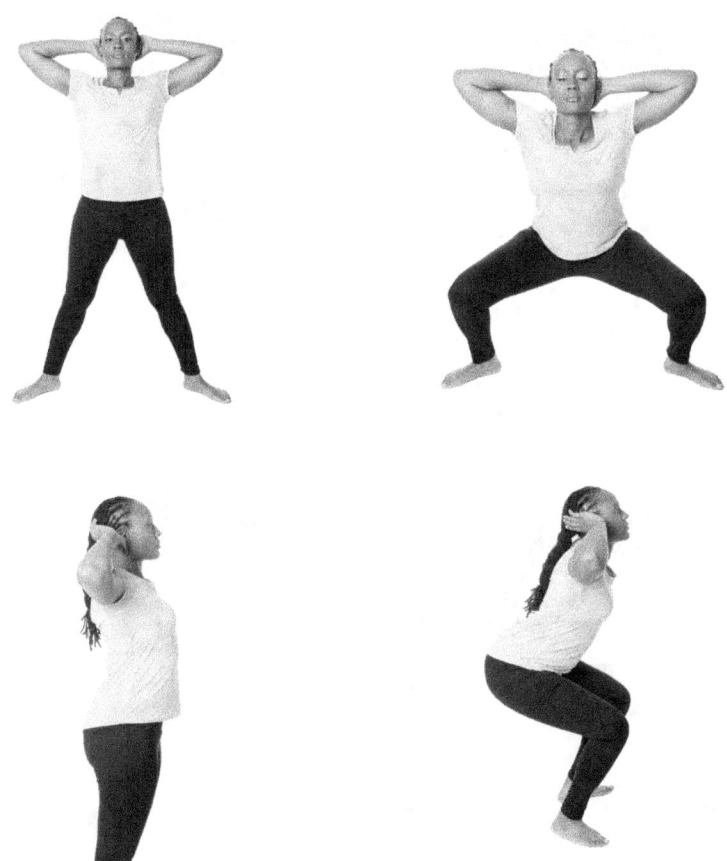

Standing Lunges: Step with your right foot forward, now squat downward, keeping your back straight, until your right knee is at a 90-degree angle. Stand up, bringing your feet together. Now step forward with your left foot, squat downward until your left knee is at a 90-degree angle. Do three sets of ten to fifteen repetitions on each leg. Note: your knee should NOT go over your toe line. Your knee should be aligned with your ankle.

Leg Curls with Physio Ball: Lying on your back place the ball under your foot/ankle. Now, bend your knees bringing the ball towards your buttocks. Do three sets of ten to fifteen repetitions.

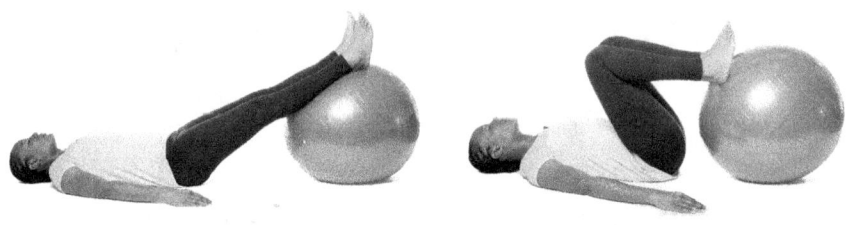

Table 12.4 Advanced Program for the Sacrum and Pelvis	
Sacrum and Pelvis Stretches	**Sacrum and Pelvis Exercises**
• See Beginner and Intermediate Sacrum and Pelvis Programs.	• Squats with Physio Ball • Sumo Squats (with or without Physio Ball) • Standing Lunges • Leg Curls with Physio Ball

	Beginner Exercise Program	Intermediate Exercise Program	Advanced Exercise Program
For:	• Individuals who just acquired an injury. • Individuals experiencing acute pain. • Experiencing exacerbation of pain or flare-up • Individuals who feel 0-29% better.	• Individual who suffer from chronic pain • Individuals who feel at least 30-50% better.	• Individuals who feel at least 80-100% better.
Cervical Spine (Neck)	*Stretches* • Ear-to-Shoulder • Head Rotation • Head Nod • 4-Point Stretch *Exercises* • Cervical Extension • Neck Push-1 • Neck Push-2	*Stretches* • Perform stretches from *Beginner Exercise Program* *Exercises* • Cervical Extension with Resistance Bands • Cervical Extension with Physio Ball • Lateral Flexion with Resistance Bands • Lateral Flexion with Physio Ball • Forward Flexion with Physio Ball	*Stretches* • Perform stretches from *Beginner Exercise Program* • Star Gaze *Exercises* • Cervical Extension (against gravity)
Thoracic Spine (Mid-Back)	*Stretches* • Hug • Hug-and-Tuck *Exercises* • Shoulder Shrugs • Shrug-and-Hold • Shoulder Blade Squeeze • Peacock	*Stretches* • Perform stretches from *Beginner Exercise Program* *Exercises* • The Crow • Rear Hand Clap • Scapular Retraction with Resistance Bands	*Stretches* • Perform stretches from *Beginer Exercise Program* *Exercises* • The Crow with Dumbbells (on Physio Ball) • Scapular Retraction with Dumbbells (on Physio Ball or wobble board) • Shoulder Shrugs with Dumbbells (seated, standing or on Physio Ball or wobble board)

Lumbar Spine (Low Back)	*Stretches* • Knee-to-Chest 1 • Knee-to-Chest 2 • Knee-to-Chest 3 *Exercises* • Abdominal Hallowing • Pelvic Lift	*Stretches* • Perform stretches from *Beginner Exercise Program* • Lumbar Twist with Physio Ball • Prayer Stretch • Cat Stretch *Exercises* • Knee-to-Chest 4 • One-Leg Bridge • Lumbar Twist • Back Extension • Modified Leg Lifts • Lef Lifts • Abdominal Crunches • Modified Low Plank • Low Plank	*Stretches* • Perform stretches from *Beginner and Intermediate Exercise programs* *Exercises* • Abdominal Crunches on Physio Ball • Back Extension on Physio Ball • High Plank • Low Plank on Physio Ball • Low Plank Elbow-Knee Touch • High Plank Elbow-Knee Touch (Opposite)
Sacrum and Pelvis	*Stretches* • Piriformis Stretch • Hamstrings Stretch • Quadriceps Stretch *Exercises* • Pelvic Rock-N-Roll with Physio Ball —Side Rock —Swoops —Clockwise Circles —Counter-Clockwise Circles	*Stretches* • Perform stretches from *Beginner Exercise Program* • Side-Lying Quadriceps Stretch • Lying Hamstring Stretch *Exercises* • Modified Side Lying Leg Lifts • Side Lying Leg Lifts • Pelvic Lift • Modified Leg Lifts • Leg Lifts • Ball Squeeze	*Stretches* • Perform stretches from *Beginner and Intermediate Exercise programs* *Exercises* • Squat with Physio Ball • Sumo Squats (with or without Physio Ball) • Standing Lunges • Leg Curl with Physio Ball

You Should Know:

- To make it more challenging by increasing the number of repetitions.
- Advance to the Elite Program if you want to increase muscle strength, gain muscle endurance and increase muscle mass.

Chapter 13

Elite Program

"I make sure I do my best, because it is always worth it, no matter what you want to achieve in life."

Andreia Brazier

The more active you are involved in your recovery the better the outcome. Take charge of your health and take full responsibility for the outcome. It is not up to the doctor to heal you, we are here to assist and guide you in any way that we can. It is up to you to heal yourself. I know, it sounds strange to say, but this is the truth. Healing does not begin from the outside it starts from within.

The Elite Program is designed for those individuals who want to continue to stay healthy and strong. This program primarily targets muscles of the back and secondarily trains the muscles of the upper extremity (e.g. biceps, triceps, and deltoids). The exercises herein will require the use of exercise equipment, such as a physio ball, wobble board or medicine ball, a pull-up bar, dumbbells and gliders. There are two routines you can choose from: the At Home Back Workout for those who do not have access to a gym and the Gym Back Workout, for those who do have access to a gym.

I encourage you to continue to perform the stretches mentioned in the Beginner and Intermediate Programs to maintain and improve spinal flexibility. The exercises in this program help improve muscle strength and endurance. If you desire to improve muscles mass then you would have to maximize your efforts by increasing the amount of resistance (e.g. the weight) and decrease the amount of repetitions.

Abdominal Exercises for Home and/or Gym
These exercises can be performed whether you follow the At Home Back Workout or the Gym Back Workout.

Dead-Man Sit-Up: Lying on your back with your arms by your side and legs straight. Now sit straight up. Do three sets of fifteen to thirty repetitions.

High Plank on Physio Ball or Medicine Ball: Start with your hands on the ball with your elbows tucked in at your side. Lift your body off the ball and hold in this position for thirty to sixty count or seconds. Perform three sets.

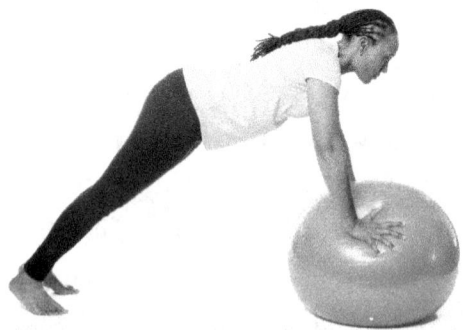

High Plank Elbow Knee Touch (on Physio Ball): Start with your hands on the ball with your elbows tucked in at your side.

Lift your body off the ball and hold in this position. Alternate bringing the knee toward the elbow on the same side. Do three sets of thirty repetitions.

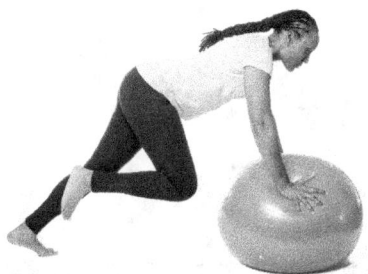

High Plank Elbow Knee Touch (on Physio Ball) (Opposite): Start with your hands on the ball with your elbows tucked in at your side. Lift your body off the ball and hold in this position. Alternate bringing the opposite knee toward the opposite elbow (e.g. right knee towards the left elbow). Do three sets of thirty repetitions.

Reverse Crunch with Gliders: Start in the high plank position with the gliders under your feet. Bring both knees up towards your elbows. Do three sets of fifteen to thirty repetitions.

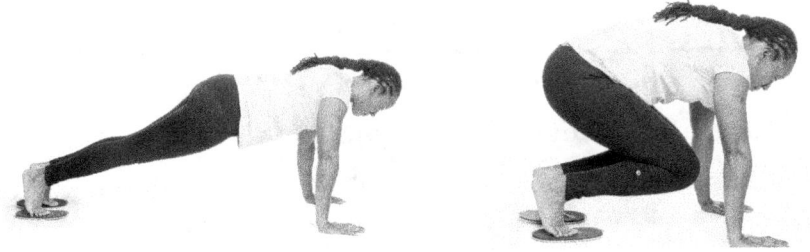

Mountain Climbers with Gliders: Start in the high plank position with the gliders under your feet. Alternate bringing your knees up toward your chest. Do three sets of fifteen to thirty repetitions.

Pikes with Physio Ball: Start in the high plank position with the ball under your feet. Keeping your knees straight, bring the ball toward your chest. Do three sets of ten to fifteen repetitions.

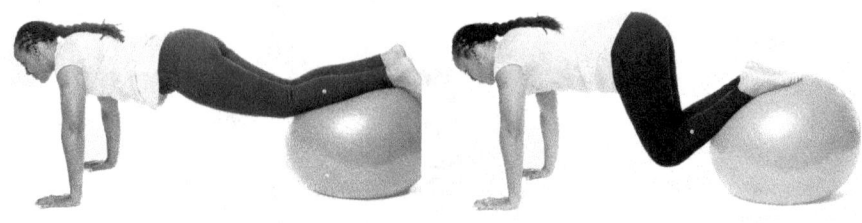

Table 13.1 Abdominal Exercises	
Exercise	Number of Repetitions/Number of Sets
Dead-Man Sit-Up	15-30 repetitions, 3 sets
High Plank on Physio Ball or Medicine Ball	Hold for 30-60 count or seconds, 3 sets
High Plank Elbow-Knee Touch (on Physio Ball) High Plank Elbow-Knee Touch Opposite (on Physio Ball)	30 repetitions, 3 sets
Reverse Crunch with Gliders	15-30 repetitions, 3 sets
Mountain Climbers with Gliders	30 repetitions, 3 sets
Pikes with Physio Ball	10-15 repetitions, 3 sets

Back Exercises for Home and/or Gym

To perform the home workout you will need the following exercise equipment: physio ball, medicine ball, pull-up bar, dumbbells, and gliders, which can be purchased from a local sporting goods store or by visiting my website, *www.drtiffanybutler.com*. Due to the fact that you are using weights, the exercises can be performed every other day to allow healing and repair of the muscle tissues. Resting in between workouts will ensure that you do not injure or damage the muscles tissues. This only includes a few exercises to get you started. There are many exercises to choose from, but the ones mentioned here are what I believe are most effective when performed properly. The exercises will be listed based on which muscle group is targeted.

Allow proper rest in between each set to bring nutrients and oxygenated blood to your muscles, so you can recover. Rest for thirty to one hundred twenty seconds between each set, depending on the amount of effort you put forth. For example, if you are working on muscle endurance then rest for thirty to sixty seconds and if you want muscle mass then rest longer (two to three minutes). Drink plenty of water. Remember, to always listen to your body. Although you do want to push yourself; however, if you feel pain and/or discomfort, stop.

Table 13.2 Extrinsic Back Muscles		
At Home Back Workout	**Gym Back Workout**	**Muscles Involved**
• Dumbbell Shrugs • Shrugs with Resistance.	• Dumbbell Shrugs • Barbell Shrugs • Cable Shrugs	• Trapezius (upper and middle fibers) • Levator scapulae
• Reverse Dumbbell Flies • Dumbbell Bent Over Row	• Reverse Dumbbell Flies • Reverse Cable Flies • Scapular Retraction with Rope • Dumbbell Bent Over Row • Barbell Bent Over Row	• Trapezius (lower fibers) • Rhomboids (major and minor) • *Posterior Deltoid*
• Pull-ups • Dumbbell Pullover	• Pull-ups • Lat. Pull Down (wide grip) • Lat. Pull Down (one arm) • One Arm Wipes • Dumbbell Pullover • Barbell Pullover	• Latissimus Dorsi • Trapezius (lower fibers) • *Biceps*

Note: AVOID doing the exercise Upright Rows to work the trapezius. This movement creates shoulder impingement syndrome, which can lead to shoulder pain.

Table 13.3 Intrinsic Back Muscles		
At Home Back Workout	**Gym Back Workout**	**Muscles Involved**
• Neck Extensions with Resistance Bands • Neck Side Flexion with Resistance Bands	• Weighted Neck Extensions • Weighted Neck Side Flexion	• Splenius capitis • Splenius cervicis • Erector Spinae • Sub occipital
• Back Extensions on Physio Ball Dumbbell Dead-lift	• Back Extensions • Low Row • Barbell Dead-lift • Good Mornings	• Erector Spinae • Semispinalis

Note: When performing the Dead-lift exercises it is important to maintain proper form and technique. Keep your back straight. Bending at the knees lift with your legs and not with your back. AVOID rounding your back; this will make you vulnerable for injury. Keep the weight as close to your legs as possible (touching your legs would be best). The further the weight is away from your body, the more pressure and strain placed on your lower back which increases your risk of injury.

The amount of repetitions and sets depend on what your goals are. See Table 13.4 for suggestions.

Table 13.4 Physical Goals		
Goal	**Strength and Endurance**	**Increase Mass**
Number of Repetitions	10-15 seconds	3-6
Number of Sets	3-4	3-6
Rest Period	30-60 seconds	60-180 seconds
Weight	Light to moderate	Moderate to heavy

When an exercise becomes easier to perform make it more challenging by doing one of the following:

- Decrease resting period.
- Increase weight.
- Increase number of sets.
- Increase number of repetitions per set.

Switch up your workout routines to create muscles confusion. The muscles are very good at adapting to new movements and they create what we call muscles memory. By changing up exercises, this creates new movement patterns and the muscles will begin to grow and get stronger.

You Should Know:

- Strength and flexibility are important in reducing our chances of injury.
- Challenge yourself by trying new exercises.
- Don't be afraid to push yourself. Muscle growth will only happen when you go against resistance.
- Despite its popularity in the body building world, Upright Rows and Lat. Pull-Down performed behind the back, increases your chance of shoulder impingement syndrome which will result in shoulder pain.

At Home Back Workout	Gym Back Workout
Back Exercises • Dumbbell Shrugs • Shrugs with Resistance Bands • Reverse Dumbbell Flies • Pull-ups • Dumbbell Pullover • Neck Extension with Resistance Bands • Neck Side Flexion with Resistance Bands • Back Extension on Physio Ball • Dumbbell Dead-lift	*Back Exercises* • Dumbbell Shrugs • Barbell Shrugs • Cable Shrugs • Reverse Dumbbell Flies • Reverse Cable Flies • Scapular Retraction with Rope • Dumbbell Bent Over Row • Barbell Bent Over Row • Pull-ups • Lat. Pull Down (wide grip) • Lat. Pull Down (one arm) • One Arm Wipes • Dumbbell Pullover • Barbell Pullover • Weighted Neck Extensions • Weighted Neck Side Flexion • Back Extensions • Low Row • Barbell Dead-lift • Good Mornings

Abdominal Exercises
- Dead-Man Sit-Up
- High Plank on Physio Ball
- High Plank Elbow-Knee Touch on Physio Ball
- High Plank Elbow-Knee Touch Opposite on Physio Ball
- Mountain Climbers with Gliders
- Pikes with Physio Ball

Phase IV

Preventing Back Pain While at Work

"Prevention is better than cure."

Desiderius Eramus

Introduction to Phase IV

Your occupation could contribute to your back pain. Think about it. If you work at a job that requires constant lifting, twisting, bending and stooping, wouldn't you experience some kind of discomfort at the end of the shift? Those whose jobs require prolong sitting such as bus operators and truck drivers are more likely to experience neck, back and leg pain. This section is to give you some practices you can put into place that will help decrease your risk of acquiring an injury while at work. Although there is no fool proof solution to totally preventing neck and back injuries at work, knowing how to reduce your chances of injury is a good start.

Chapter 14

Proper Lifting and Carrying

Lift with your legs and NOT with your back!

It is very important to lift properly, especially when carrying a load. Although most jobs are required by law to have their employees undergo work safety training, this does not, unfortunately, stop injuries all together. However, with proper training, you can reduce your risk of getting injured in the first place. Lifting is one of the common causes of back injury at work, mainly repetitive lifting, which we call microtrauma. For example, over-time doing the same motion continuously such as lifting fifty-pound boxes and loading them on a belt can fatigue the back muscles. As mentioned before in Phase I, we are more likely to injury ourselves when we are fatigued.

Therefore, lifting properly can help reduce your chance of injuring your back and missing workdays. It is reported by the Bureau of Labor Statistic more than one million workers suffer from back injuries each year. If not treated properly back injury can lead to permanent disability.

How to Lift Properly
Prior to lifting, especially something heavy, ensure that your body is

squared and centered with the object. When lifting from the floor, bend at the knees keeping your back straight, grab the object and stand up as illustrated in the picture below. This position allows you to utilize your legs to lift the load. Your back is straight and the muscles are contracted and able to handle the additional load. Thus, reducing your chance of injuring your back.

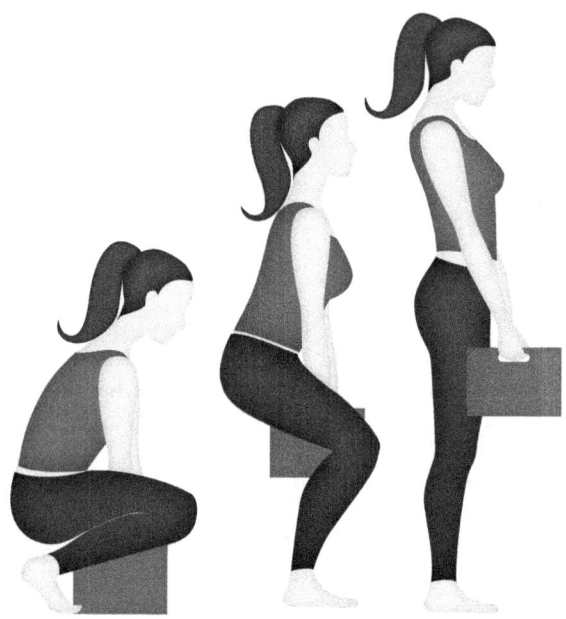

Avoid lifting with your back. Most people will not bend at the knees but at the waist, putting them more at risk for an injury. When you do this, your spinal joints are open and are not supported by the muscles because they are lengthened and stretched, as illustrated in the picture below. As you stand up, the body is not prepared to receive the additional load as a result the muscles are strained or overstretched. Although you may not feel discomfort the first few times you do this, you will experience pain and discomfort hours later.

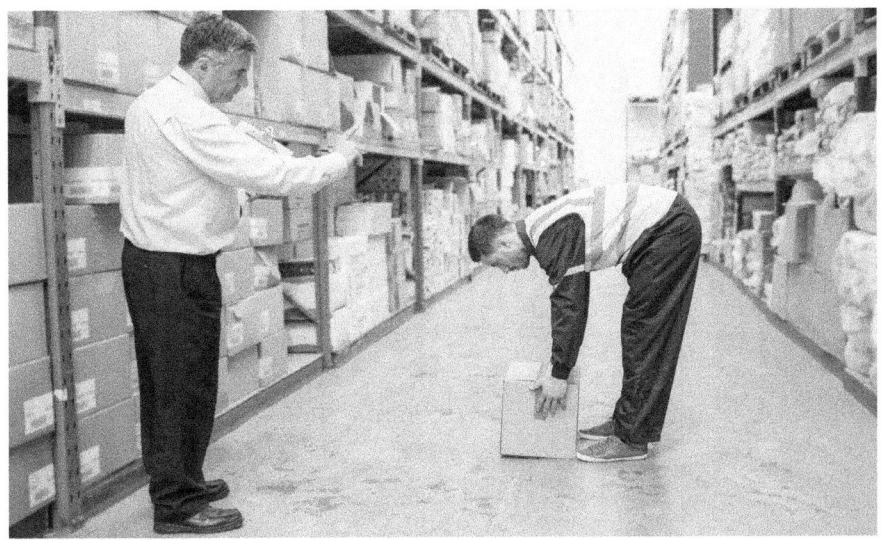

Carrying Heavy Objects

After lifting the object properly, keep it close to your body by bending your elbows in tucking them to your side. The closer it is to your body, the less work and strain on your back muscles as illustrated in the picture below.

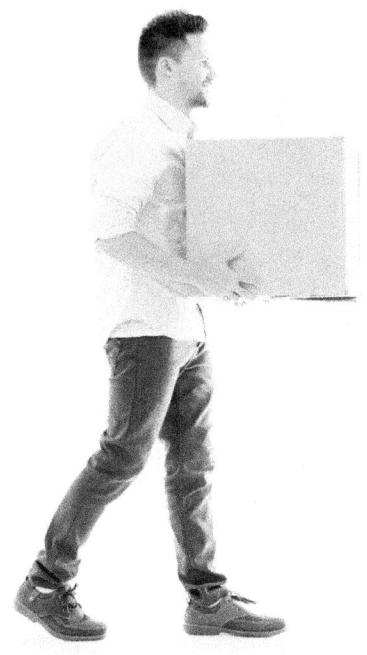

The further the object is away from your body, as demonstrated in the picture below. The more stress you place on your back muscles, resulting in them working hard, eventually they will fatigue and fail, which results in a back injury, such as a strain. Ask for help if an object is too heavy. Don't let your ego stop you from getting assistance. A back injury is far worse than a damaged ego.

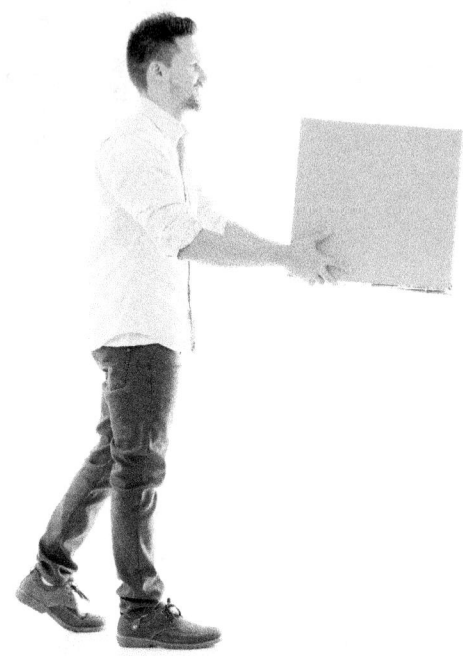

You Should Know:
- Keep your back straight and lift with your legs, NOT with your back.
- Bend at the knees and not at the waist.
- Carry objects close to your body.
- Ask for help carrying heavy objects.

Chapter 15

Work Ergonomics

We spend a third of our day working or doing work-related activities. Your occupation can contribute to your neck and back pain.

Repetitive Lifting, Twisting, Stooping, or Carrying

Occupations: warehouse, delivery, carpenter, plumber, electrician, and HVAC technician

At Risk for: neck pain, back pain, back injury, and over-use injuries

Occupations that require various body positions while performing task can increase your risk of injury. In addition, to carrying or lifting a load, repetitively doing these activities, such as twisting while carrying a load, increases your chance of injury. While lifting keep your body centered with the object. Bend at the knees and squat down, using your legs to lift the weight. Carry the object close to your body as mentioned in the previous chapter.

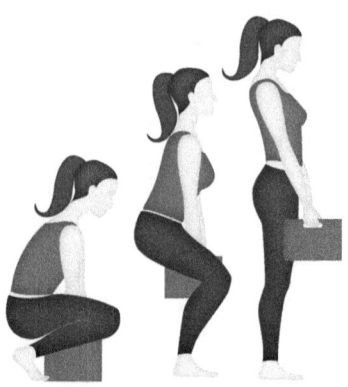

Prolong Sitting (three hours or more)

Occupation: bus operator, truck driver, and clerical and administrative

At Risk for: neck pain, back pain, poor posture, tension headache, and over-use injuries (such as Carpel Tunnel).

Those who sit more while at work have a tendency to experience tension headaches, neck and upper back pain as a result of tight neck and upper back muscles. As well as tight hamstrings and hip flexors which can contribute to lower back pain. While sitting, we alternate between sitting up straight and slouching. As our body begins to fatigue, we tend to lean forward into a flexed position; our head moves forward and our shoulders round, obtaining what I like to call a gremlin posture as illustrated in the picture below.

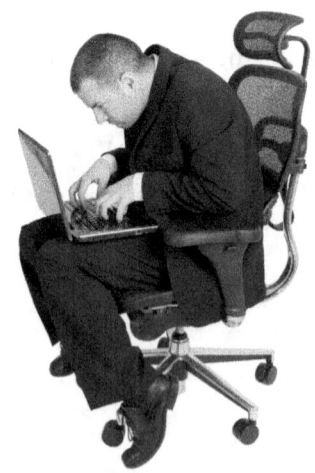

To avoid putting strain on your neck and back muscles, use a chair that provides lumbar support. Sit in the chair with your elbows, knees and hips at a 90-degree angle. Use of a physio ball can help strengthen your back muscles while sitting. Avoid slouching if possible, if you start to get tired or fatigue, take a break, get up and walk around then sit back down.

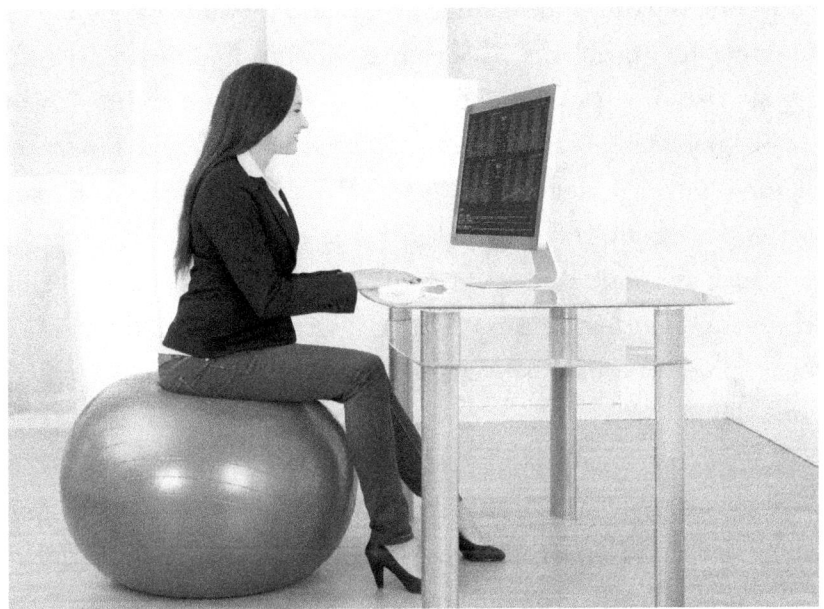

When using a desktop or laptop, ensure that the center of the computer screen is placed at eye level. Raise the computer monitor above eye-level this will force you to put your head in a slight extension position.. When using a laptop, don't actually put the laptop on your lap. This will cause your head to be in a constant flexed position, which places strain on your neck and upper back muscles. Instead, place the laptop on the table with books placed underneath and use a wireless keyboard and mouse. The monitor should be placed at or above eye level.

Take a five-minute break every hour, if possible, to go for a short walk or to simply stretch. This will get the blood circulating and loosen up any muscles that are getting tight.

Prolong Standing or Walking (three hours or more)

Occupation: cashier, retail, restaurant worker, mail carrier and security officer

At Risk for: back pain, neck pain, foot/ankle problems, varicose veins and over-use injuries such as Carpel Tunnel.

Prolong walking and standing can lead to foot/ankle problems, venous circulatory problems, back pain and joint pain. One way of reducing your risk of back pain and injury is by strength training, which increase your muscle strength and endurance allowing you to stand or walk for a longer period of time before your muscles start to fatigue.

If you are required to stand in a one place for more than three hours, such as a cashier, place a small box underneath one foot. Doing so relieves pressure off the lower back, by stretching and flattening the lumbar spine. Alternate between legs, to avoid putting more pressure on one side.

During your breaks, stretch your back and leg muscles to relax and reduce muscle tension. Make sure you are wearing shoes that support your arches and avoid wearing flats, flip-flops, sandals, and high heels. Shoes such as flip-flops, sandals and high heels, if worn for prolong hours, can lead to foot/ankle problems, as well as a back pain.

If you suffered from a recent injury to the lower back, then wearing a back brace will provide support to your back muscles and provide temporary relief while standing and/or walking. However, I would only suggest wearing the brace only while at work to prevent your body from getting use to the outside support. Remove the back brace while at home and following the Beginner Program for the Lumbar Spine to start strengthening your lower back muscles.

You Should Know:

- Carry a load close to your body to prevent strain on your lower back.

- Place the computer screen at or above eye level to reduce neck pain.
- Take a break to stretch the muscles to reduce muscle tension and tightness.
- Place a small box underneath one foot to relieve lower back tension.
- Wear a back brace or lumbar (low back) support only when you are at work or out and about, such as running errands.

Chapter 16

What to Do if I Am Injured at Work

The sooner you get help the better off you will be.

Inform Your Supervisor

If you are injured at work you may be entitled to workers' compensation, which is there to cover any medical expenses you may accumulate as a result of an on-the-job injury. If you prolong informing your supervisor, this may create problems in the future. It is best to let them know, even if you are not feeling pain and/or you think you are not hurt (injured). Your supervisor will generally make a report of the incident. Ensure that you request a copy for your personal records.

Workers' Compensation

There are federal laws in place that require most employees to have workers' compensation insurance. After reviewing your incident, they will determine whether the employer's negligence caused the injury (such as an unsafe work environment, etc.). However, if you were at fault, such as intoxicated or not wearing the proper safety equipment, you may not be entitled to coverage.

See a Doctor

Go to the emergency room if you suffered a severe injury. If you are not seriously injured then see a doctor as soon as you leave work. After examining you the doctor will instruct you on how to take care of your injuries and recommend you for treatment if necessary. Your employer may have a company doctor that you must see after an on-the-job injury; however, if you are not satisfied with the doctor, you have a right to see any healthcare professional.

If workers' compensation will not pay for your doctor's visit, then I would recommend that you seek another doctor using your health insurance. Remember it is your health, and you want to make sure that you get examined after the injury. Whether your employer will cover the expense or not.

Get Treatment

If you have suffered from an injury that requires treatment, do not delay treatment. If you have missed work because of an injury then you should be under doctor's care. I have seen many people who suffered injuries in motor vehicle accidents, who delayed treatment, and appear in my office a month later because of residual pain. An acute injury can become a chronic issue, if not treated properly. An active rehabilitative program is what you will need to overcome an injury which should incorporate therapeutic exercise and stretching.

Consult with an Attorney

You may need to consult with an attorney to determine what benefits you are entitled to receive under workers' compensation such as paid medical expenses and loss wages.

You Should Know:

- Report injury to your supervisor.

- Get a copy of the incident report.
- See a doctor to be on the safe side.
- Get treated.
- Consult with an attorney (if necessary).

Chapter 17

Maximize Your Lunch Break

Instead of eating and sitting around until the whistle blows, go for a short walk, take a nap, or attend an exercise class. When I worked for high-volume office, we would get an hour and half for lunch, which I thought was too long, but I used that time to do things. Since it only take me about ten to fifteen minutes to eat, I would go for a short walk, go to the gym, catch up on my reading or do errands. There are plenty of things you can do during your lunch break that can be beneficial to your health. I will discuss a few that are not only helpful to reducing neck and back pain but great for your overall health and wellbeing.

Perform Stretches and/or Exercises
Stretching helps improve muscle elasticity and joint flexibility. Both help with injury prevention, which allows your muscles and joints to go greater lengths before damage will occur. Exercise, especially against resistance, helps builds muscle strength and endurance. Strength and endurance allows your muscles to be able to work longer without fatiguing too quickly. Remember, when we are fatigued we are more at risk for injury. You don't need weights or a gym to perform exercise.

Refer to Phase III, which contains stretches and exercises that can be done at home or in the office.

Some Benefits of Stretching and Exercising

- Decrease risk of injury.
- Reduce health risks, including hypertension, diabetes, certain cancers, and heart disease.
- Increase circulation.
- Reduce soreness, muscles tension and spasm.
- Improve joint flexibility.
- Increase range of motion.
- Reduce stress.
- Alleviate pain.

Go for a Walk

There are many benefits of regular stretching and exercising. After eating your lunch, go for a thirty-minute walk around the block. Use this time to reflect on the good things that are happening in your life, such as a how good it is to be able to earn a living. Grab your music or bring along a friend/coworker and hit the streets. This will get your blood flowing, which carries oxygen and nutrients to your tissues.

Some Benefits of Walking

- Lose/maintain weight.
- Activate your immune system.
- Reduce health risks, including hypertension, diabetes, certain cancers, and heart disease.
- Lower your blood pressure.
- Regulate blood sugar.
- Elevate your mood.
- Get more energy.

Take a Power Nap

Do you remember taking a nap in school right after recess? Ah, those were the good old days. In a society that is driven by deadlines, we often times become overstressed, over-worked and burnt out. Work should be enjoyable. Our bodies manifest stress in different forms of diseases, such as hypertension, diabetes, neck pain, back pain, joint pain, headaches, etc.

Taking a nap in the middle of the day is not as uncommon as you think. Simply resting for about twenty to thirty minutes can leave you recharged, relaxed and ready to conquer the second half of the day.

Some Benefits of Taking a Power Nap

- Restore/Increase alertness.
- Relaxation.
- Improved mood.
- Improved performance.

Prayer/Meditation

One of the easiest ways to change your mood is by simply expressing gratitude and appreciation for what you do have. Regardless of what you are dealing with at the current moment, there is always someone who is dealing with something worse and your situation could be worse. Take a few moments throughout the day to reflect on what you do have and avoid focusing on what you do not have. When we do this, we open up our minds to all possibilities.

Some Benefits of Prayer/Meditation

- Decrease blood pressure.
- Decrease anxiety/stress.
- Deeper spiritual connection.
- Positive outlook.
- Lower resting heart rate.

Attend a Treatment Session

If your injury requires treatment, then utilizing your lunch break to attend treatment is a good idea. You will generally avoid the morning and evening crowds. Don't delay getting treatment especially if you need it. The worst thing you can do is put off treatment; by doing so, the condition can possibly become worse. Remember, your body begins to heal immediately, therefore doing things that will aid and speed the healing process would be to your advantage.

Some Benefits of Getting Treatment

- Speed the healing process.
- Get back to work soon.
- Avoid missing days from work.
- Return to normal activities sooner.
- Increase function.
- Relieve symptoms such as pain.
- Improve range of motion.
- Provide emotional boost.

You Should Know:

- Perform stretches and/or exercise during your breaks to relieve muscle tension.
- Go for a walk to boost your mood.
- Take a power nap to increase your energy.
- Pray or meditate to gain a positive outlook.
- Attend a treatment session to relieve your symptoms.

Phase V

Preventing Back Pain at Home

"Nature performs the cure, the physician takes the fee."
Benjamin Franklin

Introduction to Phase V

Being actively involved in your health and recovery is very important. Preventing neck and back pain by avoiding activities that would increase your risk of injury and/or exacerbate your current symptoms are necessary. Certain daily activities over a period of time can lead to unwanted pain and discomfort. Activities such as texting and sleeping on an old lumpy mattress can be the cause of your headaches, neck and back pain.

Chapter 18
Sleep like a Baby

"Sleep is that golden chain that ties health and our bodies together."
Thomas Dekker

Waking Up with Back Pain: The Mattress Could Be the Culprit
We spend a third of our lives sleeping. Although most researchers do not know exactly why we sleep; however it is concluded that if we are sleep deprived we have a decline in our overall health and function. Therefore, if we spend most of our lives in bed, we should invest in a mattress that is comfortable for our bodies that will allows us the get the quality sleep we deserve.

Our bodies are constantly working throughout the day regulating our heart rate, blood sugar, fighting off diseases and infections. Sleeping plays an important role in repairing our bodies from the everyday wear and tear. Human growth hormone (HGH) plays an important role in protein production, tissue repair and metabolism. A large amount of HGH is released during the hours of 10 P.M. to 2 A.M. So if you are a night owl, you are not getting the full benefits of this important hormone. Quality sleep should have you feeling charged, refreshed and ready to take on the new day.

If you spend most of the night tossing and turning or you wake up with neck and/or back pain the culprit maybe your mattress and/or pillow.

Invest in a Good Mattress

If you're not getting enough sleep it may be time to purchase a new mattress. Find a mattress that is comfortable to you. Firm, soft or medium there are many to choose from. When shopping for a mattress shop around for the best deal, test the mattress before purchasing and get advice from a chiropractor if necessary. Although chiropractors are not sleep experts, we can advise.

When Should You Get a New Mattress?
- If you wake up with neck and/or back pain.
- If you wake up with headaches.
- If you toss and turn throughout the night.
- If you wake up tired or sleepy.
- If the mattress is lumpy, saggy and old.

When selecting a new mattress remember you are going for personal comfort.

Tips for Selecting a Mattress
- Go to a mattress store they have a wider selection to choose from.
- Lay on the mattress for about fifteen minutes.
- For couples, really consider purchasing a bed that allows individual comfort control, such as the Sleep Number Bed. It is possible that what may be considered comfortable for you can be miserable for your partner.

Waking Up with a Stiff Neck: The Pillow Could Be the Culprit
A Good Pillow

The average adult head weighs between ten to twelve pounds; over time those nice fluffy pillows will turn into flat pancakes. If you wake up with a headache, neck, mid or upper back pain, your pillow maybe the culprit. The pillow is meant to provide support to the cervical spine; however, many people sleep with too many pillows, flat pillows or no pillow at all. Although your body is essentially at rest while sleeping, using too many pillows or no pillow can create unnecessary strain on the neck muscles.

You want to have a pillow that supports your neck regardless of what type of sleeping position you are in. In the section Sleeping Positions, I discuss the best positions to minimize strain on the neck and back. Pillows do not last forever and should be replaced one to two years depending on the amount of wear and tear.

When to Get New Pillows
- Pillow is flat.
- Pillow has lost its springiness.
- If you wake up with headaches.
- If you wake up with neck pain.
- If you wake up with upper back or mid-back pain.

A Good Night's Sleep Does a Body Good

While sleeping our bodies release chemicals and hormones, such as growth hormone that plays an important role in tissue repair, cell reproduction and regeneration, stimulation of the immune system as well as other bodily functions. It is not how long you sleep, but the quality of sleep you get. The amount of sleep varies from person to person. Some people can function getting only four hours of sleep while others need eight hours to feel refreshed. Regardless of what your magic number is, getting regular sleep helps us stay healthy and improve our function.

Some Benefits of Quality Sleep
- Restore/Improve alertness.
- Improve your mood.
- Improve immune function.
- Improve memory and learning.
- Reduces stress.
- Allows body to repair from.
- Improve energy.

Sleeping Positions

Your sleeping position can possibly contribute to waking up with neck and/or back pain. Ideally, when you are sleeping you want your body to be in a neutral position. When we sleep, we really do not have control over our bodies. We toss and turn, and wonder how we end up lying side-ways with the covers and pillows on the floor. By sleeping in a neutral position, especially if you are experiencing neck and/or back pain, will alleviate strain on your neck and back muscles.

Back Sleeper

Sleeping in is this position doesn't normally put unnecessary strain on the neck and/or back muscles. A good pillow should be placed in the center of the head. This position provides support to the neck by keeping the spine in a neutral position, which will help to relieve neck pain. Resting your head on fluffy pillows or too many pillows in this position can cause headaches, neck, upper and/or mid back pain. Sleeping with too many pillows or a big fluffy pillow puts your neck in a flexed position with your chin tucked. This position stretches the posterior neck muscles and you may experience pain if held in this position for more than thirty minutes.

By placing a pillow under your knees, this will help flatten the lumbar spine relieving pain to the lower back.

Side Sleeper or Fetal Position

This is the most common sleeping position, the Side Sleeper or Fetal position, especially in women. This maybe because we spend the first nine months of our lives in the fetal position in the womb and perhaps the position that we are most comfortable and reminds us of a safe place. To avoid waking up with neck or back pain, keep the spine in a neutral position. If you are experiencing neck pain, avoid sleeping with too many pillows or a big fluffy pillow which puts your head in a side flexed position. This position stretches the lateral (side) neck muscles and more than likely you will experience neck pain and/or discomfort if held in this position for more than thirty minutes. Sleeping with no pillow or a flat pillow does the same as mentioned above, but on the opposite side of the neck.

If you are experiencing low back pain, sleeping with a pillow between your knees will help prevent you from twisting, which can place strain on the lower back.

Stomach Sleeper

This position can place strain on the neck and back muscles. If you are experiencing neck, mid and/or upper back pain, try to avoid this position. Sleeping on your stomach forces you to turn your head to one side-which can place unwanted strain on your neck muscles.

Sleeping in this position accentuates the lower back curve, placing more strain on the low back muscles.

If you are experiencing lower back pain, place a pillow under your pelvis to help flatten your lower back, this will help alleviate back pain.

You Should Know:

- If you are awakening with neck and/or back pain, it could be your mattress or pillow.
- Select a mattress that is personally comfortable. Firm or soft doesn't always mean comfortable.
- Avoid sleeping with too many pillows or a big pillow, which can put unwanted strain on your neck and back muscles.
- Place a pillow behind your knees (Back Sleepers) or between your knees (Side Sleeper or Fetal Position) to alleviate lower back pain.
- Keep your spine in a neutral position and avoid twisting, if possible.
- Quality, not quantity, of sleep helps us stay healthy and improve our overall function.

Chapter 19
Modern Technology

*"Take a break from media and television that isn't delivering
a positive message. The input you absorb is a heavy contrib-
utor to your health, or lack of it."*

J.J. Goldwag

In the age of technology and information most of the people in the
United States have access to a computer and cell phone. Although our
lives have changed dramatically over the last twenty years our lifestyles
have changed as well.

Cell Phone Use
Talking on the Cell Phone
The days of using a phone with a wire attached to it is slowly coming to
an end. Mobile phones are the new home phones and in some cases, work
phones. It is estimated that over six billion people in the world have access
to cell phones. With the increase of cell phone use, there also has been
an increase in the number of complaints of headaches, neck pain, upper
back pain, and hand pain associated with cell phone use.

I've seen many people talk on a cell phone holding the phone between their ear and shoulder. After doing this for about ten minutes,

you will experience neck pain. However, doing this multiple times throughout the day can create tightness in the neck and upper back muscles and over time can lead to tension headaches, neck and/or upper back pain.

Some Tips on Talking on the Cell Phone

- Avoid holding the phone with your ear on your shoulder.
- Use the speaker or a hands-free device such as an earpiece.

Texting

It is estimated that the average teenager send over one hundred text messages a day compared to the average adult eighty-seven according to a study conducted by Paw Research Center. Most people will send a text message before calling it has become the norm. Not only can excessive text message cause tension headaches, neck and upper back pain it can also create pain and discomfort in the thumbs. If your neck is hurting from texting too much, then take a break. Use the phone to make an actual call. Verbal communication is essential to our existence as humans. Hearing someone say I love you and reading "I love you" will be received differently.

Some Tips When Texting

- Look up once in a while.
- Bring the phone to eye-level to avoid constant neck flexion.
- Use the phone to make a phone call. Hearing a laugh and reading laugh out loud has a different effect.

Computer Use
Desktop and Laptop

Whether you are using a desktop or a laptop, the top of the monitor should be placed at eye-level to avoid strain on the neck muscles. When using a desktop raise the monitor (if you have this function) or place books underneath the monitor, to elevate it to eye level. The longer you sit at the computer the more likely you will develop poor posture. Your eyes start to fatigue, your head goes forward to see the screen better and your upper back becomes rounded. Now you are sitting in a hunched or gremlin position that you may not be aware of. This maybe your normal sitting position, either way it is bad for your back. Sitting in this hunched position for hours a day, week after week, can lead to headaches, neck pain, back pain and possibly pain into the arms. Pay attention to your posture when using the computer. Most people have poor posture because they are simply unaware of it.

Using a laptop can cause you to sit in a hunched slouched position, which can cause neck, upper back and lower back pain. When using a laptop, place it under books or a shelf to put the screen at eye-level then use a wireless keyboard and mouse.

Take a break, if possible, every hour to avoid strain on the eyes, neck and back muscles. Performing the cervical exercises and stretches mentioned in Chapter 11: Beginner Program, will help reduce muscles tension and promote muscles relaxation.

Revisit Chapter 15: Work Ergonomics on proper body positioning when using a computer.

Some Tips When Using a Computer
- Raise the monitor/screen to eye-level to avoid neck strain.
- Use a wireless keyboard and mouse when using a laptop.

Reading and Studying
When reading or studying use a bookstand or hold the book up with your elbows bent to eye-level to avoid having your neck in a constant flexed position. Reading or studying for hours with your neck in a flexed position can create unwanted neck pain and discomfort, as well as

headaches. Take a five-minute break every hour to stretch and loosen up your muscles. This will increase blood flow to the neck and head, as well as your brain.

Some Tips for Reading and Studying
- Use a bookstand.
- Hold the book up at eye-level.
- Take a five-minute break every hour to stretch your neck muscles to reduce muscle tension.

You Should Know:
- Excessive texting can cause thumb pain, as well as neck and upper back pain.
- Elevate the computer monitor/screen to eye-level to avoid strain on the neck.
- Take a five-minute break, if possible from computer use, reading and studying, to stretch the neck muscles. This increase blood flow to the head and neck region and promote muscles relaxation.

Chapter 20
Driving

"A life that finds joy and peace to balance stress and strife will increase its opportunity for health."

J.J. Goldwag

Driving to/from Work

Most people spend an average ninety minutes a day commuting to and from work. This means a lot of sitting in the car, train and/or bus. Constant sitting can cause tight hamstrings, hip flexors, and pectorals (chest) muscles, as well as neck and back pain. To avoid experiencing neck and back pain from driving, avoid slouching. Sit with the seat in a comfortable position with your head centered against the headrest and your arms slightly bent The headrest is there for a reason, in the event of a car accident, it prevents your neck from hyper-extending and fracturing. Once your seat is positioned comfortable, adjust the mirrors.

Sit with your knees slightly bent to relax the thigh muscles. Some newer vehicles have a lumbar support control in the seat, which can provide varies amounts of pressure to support the lower back. If your car does not have this ability, then use a small pillow to give support to yyour lumbar spine. Keeping the spine in its normal position while driving will reduce the amount of strain on the neck and back muscles.

Relax when holding the steering wheel and avoid clinching or squeezing it. Doing so will lead to muscles fatigue in the hand and fore-arms. Pay attention to your posture, if you are starting to slouch then correct your seat.

Tips for Driving to/from Work

- Keep your head in the center of the headrest.
- Don't slouch. Sit in an upright comfortable position.
- Use a small pillow or lumbar pillow to support your lower back.
- Keep a slight bend in your knees and elbows to relax the thigh and arm muscles.

Long-Distance Driving

Those who spend more than 75 percent of their shift driving such as tractor trailer operators and taxi drivers are more likely to experience neck pain, back pain, as well as knee pain, from prolonged sitting and shifting the foot between the accelerator and brakes.

Long-distance driving, like prolong sitting, has been linked with an increased risk for health problems, such as obesity. In addition to the manual handling of vehicle as well as constant vibrations from the vehicle can be physically demanding.

Use a lumbar support to help maintain the lumbar curve while driving. The more natural the position of the spine, the less strain is placed on the muscles. Driving for a long distance causes the muscles, tendons and ligaments to tighten. Take breaks, if possible, to stretch the neck and back muscles, as well as the thigh muscles to reduce muscle tightness, increase blood circulation and promote relaxation.

Tips for Driving Long Distances

- Use a small pillow or lumbar pillow to maintain the natural curve of the lumbar spine.
- Take a break every two to three hours, if possible, to walk around, stretch and loosen up.
- Whether you are driving for work or for leisure, maintaining a good driving posture can reduce your chances of experiencing neck and back pain.

You Should Know:

- Make sure your head is centered to the headrest.
- Avoid slouching while driving this puts strain on the neck and back muscles.
- Sit in a comfortable position with the elbows and knees slightly bent.
- Take a break every two to three hours to stretch and relax muscles.

Phase VI

The Importance of Physical Fitness

"Physical fitness is not only one of the most important keys to a healthy body, it is the basis of dynamic and creative intellectual activity."

John F. Kennedy

Introduction to Phase VI

Physical fitness is a state of physiological well-being and the ability to perform everyday activities. It is the ability to do certain activities such as your occupation, house chores and even sports with little to no effort. For example, running a mile without being completely exhausted when you cross the finish line. Physical fitness is achieved through strength training, good nutritional intake, and proper rest. We all should aim to achieve some level of physical fitness. If our goal is to maintain a good level of physical fitness, then we will adopt a lifestyle that promotes this. By the end of this phase, you will learn why physical fitness is important in maintaining an active and healthy life.

Chapter 21

Low Impact, but Effective

"To enjoy the glow of good health, you must exercise."

Gene Tunney

Low impact exercises are not only good for your heart and lungs, but they are better for your joints. For individuals who suffer from osteoarthritis of the hip or knee joints, going for a one-mile run on the treadmill may not be a good idea. However, there are many exercises that are effective and spare the joints from constant pounding. Low impact exercises are a form of aerobic exercises in which you are using little to no resistance to perform the movement.

For those people who may suffer from back pain low impact exercises can be easier to perform and does not require the physical demands that high-impact (such as running) exercises do which places a lot of stress on the joints.

Below are some low impact exercises that if done regularly can reduce neck and back pain symptoms.

Swimming or Water Aerobics
One of the most effective activities anyone can perform for a total body

workout is swimming. The water provides an environment that reduces the amount of pressure on your joints and spine. While in the water you can perform a variety of exercises (such as squats) and the water acts as a resistance. Water therapy is an ideal exercise for those individuals who have chronic back pain and for those individuals who cannot yet perform exercises on the floor, like those mentioned in Phase III.

Cycling or Stationary Bike

Biking is another activity that reduces the amount of pressure on the hip, knee and ankle joints. Using the stationary bike is ideal for anyone who has knee and hip pain. However, if you experience back pain, biking can possibly exacerbate the pain due the seated position. Therefore use a recumbent bike instead of an upright bike to reduce the amount of strain placed on the lower back. The benefits of biking are strengthening of the lower body muscles, increase cardiovascular strength, as well as burn excess fat.

Elliptical Machine

The elliptical machine generally uses a gliding mechanism that allows you to go through motions such as running, walking or climbing. Unlike the treadmill, it places little pressure on the spine and joints. With added resistance, it can help improve muscular strength.

Walking

Walking is a great exercise. The best part is anyone can do it regardless of his or her body age. It is a great way to get the blood flowing and reduce stress. However, you don't want to walk as if you are strolling through the mall, walk with the purpose of increasing your heart rate and getting a good workout.

Benefits of Low Impact and Aerobic Exercise
- Reduce joint pain, muscle stiffness and tightness/spasm.

- Can elevate mood and decrease stress/anxiety.
- Reduce symptoms (e.g. less pain).
- Helps maintain function.
- Strengthens muscles, ligaments, and bones.
- Decrease risk of health conditions such as coronary artery disease.
- Regulate blood sugar.
- Regulate blood pressure.

The low impact exercises should be performed with a level of intensity that increases your heart rate. Your aim is to perform aerobic exercises, such as low impact exercises, at 50-85 percent of your target heart rate. Your target heart rate is about two hundred twenty minus your age. For example, a thirty-year-old woman target heart rate is one hundred ninety beats per minute. She should perform aerobic exercises at ninety-five to one hundred sixty-two beats per minute target heart rate zone. If you're not sweating you're not working hard enough. Whatever exercise you choose, perform that exercise for at least thirty minutes a day to promote overall health and wellbeing.

You Should Know:
- Low impact exercises can be very effective if done regularly.
- Low impact exercises reduce the amount of stress on your spine and joints.
- Low impact exercises are ideal for those who have chronic back pain, lower extremity joint pain (e.g. hip or knee) and the elderly.

Chapter 22

Strength and Conditioning

*"Time and health are two precious assets that we don't rec-
ognize and appreciate until they have been depleted."*

Denis Waitley

Strength Training

Endurance Requires Strength

As our bodies age it doesn't matter if we can run a 5k or climb mount
Everest, what does matter is being able to do activities of daily living
such as carrying groceries, opening jars, cooking, cleaning and groom-
ing all of which requires balance, coordination, flexibility and strength.
Research shows that muscle mass starts to decline around forty years
old and slowly continue to do so; in addition, muscle strength declines
also. To slow down this process it is not only essential to institute a
weight training program into your life, it is absolutely necessary.

Some Benefits of Strength Training
- Increase strength.
- Increase endurance.
- Increase power.

- More stamina/energy.
- Weight loss.
- Reduce risk of injury.
- Improve bodily functions (such as digestion).
- Sleep better.
- Stronger bones.
- Improve confidence and self-esteem.
- Help control blood sugar and blood pressure.
- Improve balance and coordination.

Can You Pass a Strength Test?

Looking physically strong and being physically strong are two different things. Some have the appearance of physical strength but they lack true physical power. The average person should be able to squat their body weight, however, the average person cannot because they do not train to do so. Most are misled and misguided on what to do. There is so much information found in magazines, on television, and on the Internet proclaiming to be the newest and most effective for weight loss, muscle gain, etc. Although some are effective programs and some products do work however, the majority are insufficient and ineffective.

Whether you are currently on a strength-training program or you're just getting started, knowing where you are is important. It is good to test your strength every now and again, especially if you are working towards a fitness goal. It's a good way to check progress and a way of measuring whether you need to kick it up a notch or change routines.

The Strength Tests in the Appendix Table 22.1 are used to test your core, upper body and lower body strength. Whenever I start a new weight training program, I perform the following tests to know where I am, then perform them again thirty days later to see if I have improved. The tests are a great way to track and record your progress. Take the test, record your scores and see how you measure up. See Appendix for scoring.

Perform the following exercises and record your results. The purpose of the test is to measure your body strength and endurance.

Pull-Up or Chin-Up Test: This is a test used to assess upper body strength. To perform the test, start with your arms fully extended with palms facing forward or backward. The feet must be free, not touching anything and the legs can be straight (start position). Now raise your body up by pulling up until your chin is above the bar then lower your body until your arms are fully extended (end position). No jerking, swinging or kicking allowed. This is not a timed test. Do as many pull-ups as you can before getting off the bar.

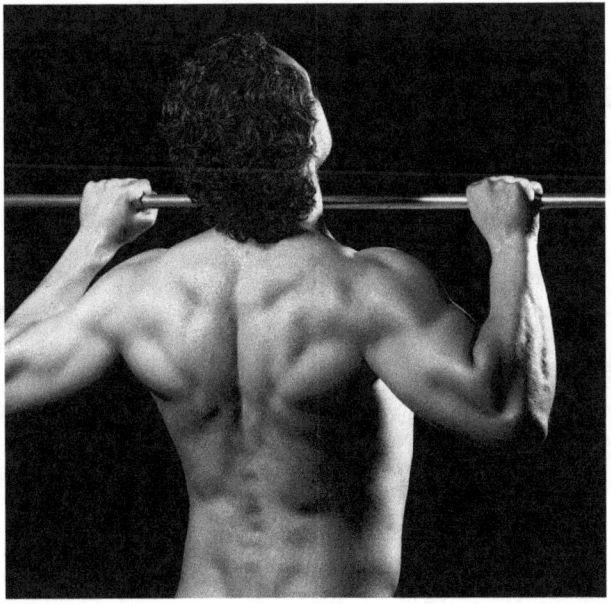

Push-Up Test: To perform the test, start with your elbows bent and by your side (start position). Now lift your body completely off the floor and extend your arms fully (end position). Avoid hiking or sagging your hips. Record how many push-ups you can perform until exhaustion. If you need to rest, rest only in the up position.

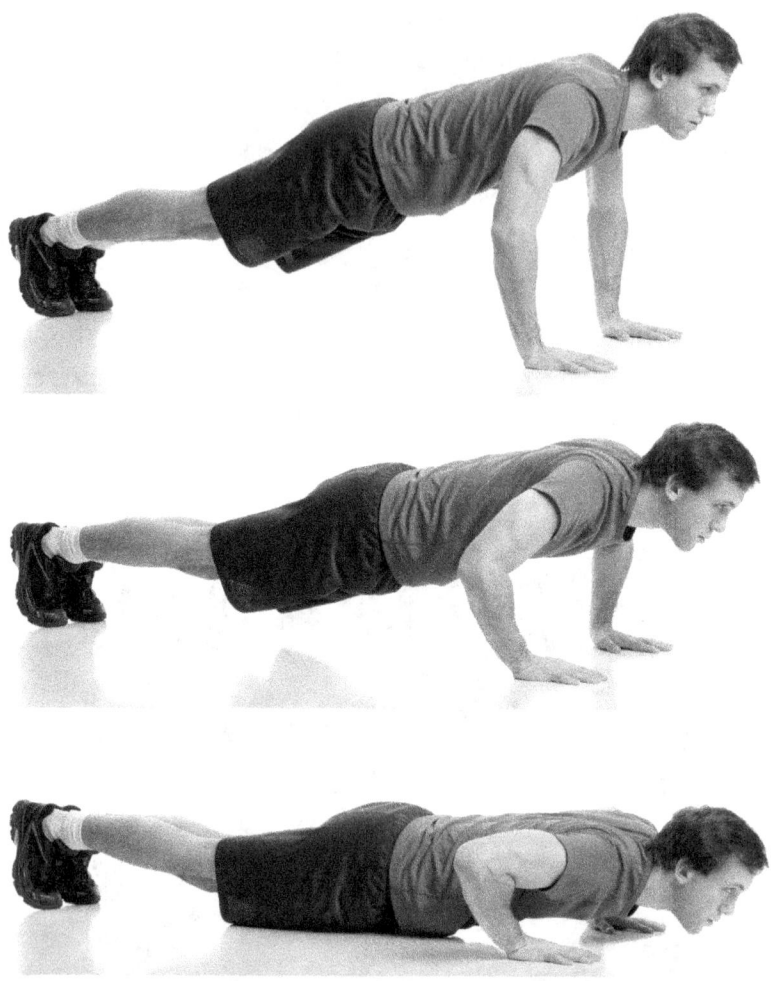

Flexed Arm Hang Test (for women or youth): This is an alternative for women to perform instead of the pull-up test. This is used to tests upper body strength, in particular back strength. To perform the test, start with your arms fully extended with palms facing forward or backward. The feet must be free, not touching anything and the legs can be straight or bent (start position). Now lift yourself up until your elbows are bent and your chin is above the bar and the body is motionless (end position). This is a timed test. Start the timer once you are in the end position. You are allowed to drop below the bar, but your elbows must maintain a flexed position. Once you drop off the bar and/or your arms are fully extended stop the timer.

One Minute Sit-up Test: This is a timed test. This is used to test abdominal strength. Lie on the floor with your knees bent, with your feet flat on the floor. Cross your arms in front your chest (start position). Now, squeeze your stomach lifting your chest towards your knees (end position). When lowering yourself, make sure your back touches the ground. Avoid tucking your chin. And, remember to breathe. Perform as many sit-ups as you can in one-minute and record the score.

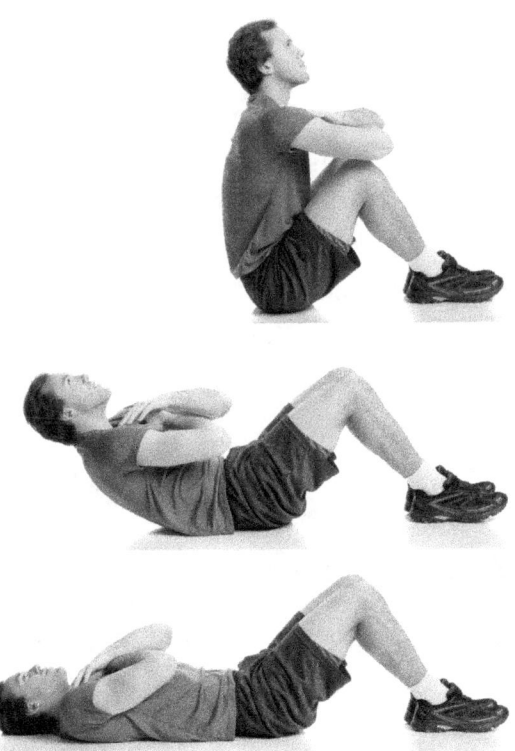

Back Extension Test: I used this test in my office to determine the strength of the intrinsic (deep back) muscles. The intrinsic muscles are used to help extend your back (bend you backward) and maintain posture. To perform this test lay on the floor face down, placing you're hands down by your side (start position). Now lift your chest and shoulders off the floor and hold this position for as long as you can. This is a timed test. Stop the timer if your chest touches the floor or if your legs come off the floor.

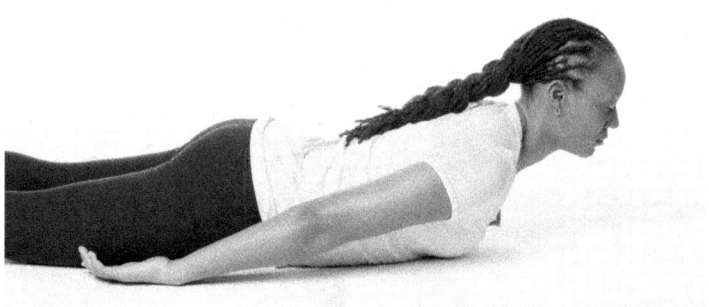

Low Plank Test: This is another test that is used to test abdominal strength. This is a timed test. To perform this test lay on the floor face down, with your elbows bent and your palms down (start position). Now lift your body off the floor and hold in this position for as long as you can. Stop the timer if you drop to the floor, your hips start to sag and/or hike.

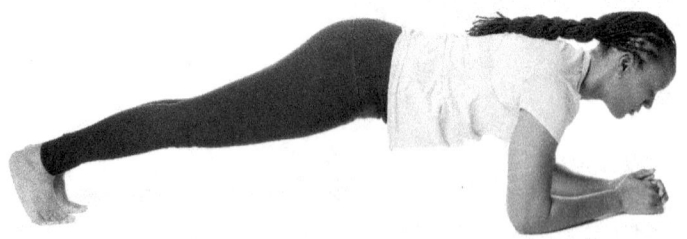

Dead-man Sit-up Test: Lie on the floor with your legs straight (start position). Now squeeze your stomach lifting your upper body off the floor, as if you were doing a sit-up. Avoid using your hands or bending your knees. This is a pass/fail test.

Squat Test: Stand in front of a chair with your feet at least shoulder width apart or whatever position is most comfortable for you with your arms folded across your chest (start position). Squat down until your buttocks lightly touch the chair with your knees at a 90-degree angle (do not sit down!), then stand straight up. This is one repetition. Do as many squats until you are exhausted.

What you do during your younger years, will manifest itself in your latter years. If you have a sedentary lifestyle, poor nutritional intake and do not exercise, it will show up later as a form of disease such as a diabetes or hypertension. To keep your strength throughout your lifetime and to maintain physical health you must have an active lifestyle, good nutritional intake and perform exercises regularly. Your exercise program should include aerobic activity, strength training and a flexibility regime which will reduce your risk of certain diseases such as heart problems, diabetes, hypertension and some cancers.

Conditioning Training
Muscle Conditioning Improves Strength and Endurance
Once you start to strengthen your muscles through resistance training then you should work towards improving your muscle endurance. Muscle conditioning is having the ability to move a muscle group (such as the leg muscles) through a specific exercise such as squats in order to improve muscle strength and endurance. Using the exercises mentioned in this book in Phase III will help you to achieve conditioning of the muscles. This can be done by performing exercises at home and/or at the gym.

Some Benefits of Conditioning Training

- Injury prevention.
- Increase strength.
- Increase endurance.
- More energy/stamina.
- Improve performance in daily activities and hobbies.
- Gain confidence.
- Increased power.
- Improve balance and coordination.
- Improve agility.
- Improved flexibility.
- Help regulate blood pressure and blood sugar.
- Bone health.
- Improved overall fitness.

Conditioning training has many benefits, not only does it improve your strength and endurance but you will be able to perform daily activities with more ease. Aerobic classes, such as Pilates, may use a combination of body-weight exercises. There are plenty of conditioning programs available to participate in, whether you attend a group session at the local gym or purchase a DVD and perform the exercises from the comfort of your own home, it has wonderful benefits. Most classes have body-weight exercises or exercises performed with weights or a combination of the two. The goal is to perform the exercises with high intensity and if done correctly on a regular basis you will see improvements.

Type of Conditioning Program/Classes

- Pilates
- Yoga
- Outdoor Cycling or Indoor Spin Class
- Boot camp

- Kickboxing
- Martial Arts (e.g. Karate, Kickboxing)
- Self-Defense
- Sports (e.g. Basketball, soccer)
- Swimming or Water Aerobics

It is never too late to improve yourself or to change. Once you reach a goal, create another one. Once you reach that one then create another. Keep doing this until the end of your days. It is very important that we have something to look forward to each and every day. The gym I frequent consist of a mixture of people, all at different stages in their lives. Maintaining a healthy way of living is not a fad, nor should it be a temporary goal. It is a lifestyle. If you go to the gym, you do it not because you simply enjoy it but because it is a part of your life. Remember, you only are given one body. Although, you can replace some parts, if they become dysfunctional because of disease, they may not always function like the original parts. Your body and all of its members were created just for you. It is important that we respect our bodies and be kind to it. Take care of your body, it's the only one you have.

You Should Know:
- Strength and conditioning is important to maintaining physical fitness.
- Activities such as cycling or swimming can help improve your muscle strength and endurance.
- Muscle endurance is a result from improved muscle strength.
- Test yourself by performing the strength tests. Remember to re-test yourself every thirty days to track and measure your progress.
- Strength, flexibility, balance, coordination, and endurance must be maintained throughout our lives.

Chapter 23

Balance, Coordination, and Flexibility

"Happiness is not a matter of intensity but of balance, order, rhythm and harmony."

Balance is important in our ever-changing environment

Have you ever walked down the street and tripped on the sidewalk, but did not fall flat on your face? Now, imagine watching a person with poor balance, shuffling along on the sidewalk, tripping on that same sidewalk. What do you think will happen to them? More than likely they will fall. Balance and coordination is not only necessary in performing thoughtless activities such as walking, driving or getting dressed, it is essential in order to perform these activities of daily living.

In order to perform exercises or to play sports, it is important to have balance and coordination. Balance is your ability to remain in an upright position or remain in a position without losing control or falling. An example of good balance would be standing with your feet together and not swaying forward, backward and/or sideways.

Exercises such as lunges and squats work on balance. While you're performing the exercise, your muscles and joints are communicating with your brain and in turn your brain signals the abdominal, back and leg muscles to contract so that you will not tip over. Balance is important because without it, we would have difficulty performing task such as walking on uneven surfaces, going up/downstairs and maintaining different body positions (posture). Therefore balance training is important as it improves coordination, posture and reduce the risk of injuries from a fall. As our body ages it is important to maintain good balance to prevent from falling which can lead to body injuries such as a fracture hip.

You can balance train by performing exercises using an unstable surface. For example, instead of doing push-ups on the floor try doing push-ups using two medicine balls. Place a medicine ball under each hand and go to work. Not only will it be more difficult and challenging to do, the benefit is that it will increase joint stability and strengthen muscles. Table 23.1 has a list of some balance exercises you can incorporate into your workout regime. There are many exercises you can perform. The exercises listed here are just to get you started. Plus, you can do them anywhere. In addition, regular practice of yoga and Tai chi can improve balance, posture, and coordination.

Start at the beginner exercises, once you have mastered those then move to the next level. The goal is to be able to perform each exercise without falling. The more you practice the better you become. To make the exercises more challenging at any level, close your eyes. We rely on three things for balance, our ears, eyes and the sensory input from the foot/ankle joints. In addition, performing the exercises barefoot will take the stability and support away that shoes provide. Thus making the foot muscles stronger.

Benefits of Training Barefoot
Our feet are the foundation and support base in which we stand and move. Therefore it is essential to have a strong base. Lack of strength, proprioception (the ability to know/sense/detect where you are in

space), and strength within the joints of the foot and ankle can make us more susceptible to injury. Wearing shoes all day can prevent the joints in our foot from moving and in a sense weaken our foot muscles because they are not working. For example, remember the last time you went to the beach, you spent hours in the sun walking around barefoot in the sand. The next day, your feet and legs were sore; this is because your foot muscles were actually working. Performing exercises such as the balance exercises barefoot will not only improve your overall balance and coordination, but will help strengthen your foot and ankle joints as well.

Coordination is required to perform voluntary actions.

Notice how easy it is for you to pick up your fork and bring food to your mouth. You do it without thinking and more than likely you do not notice all of the muscles working to do that action. The cerebellum controls balance and the coordination of movements. Although the cerebellum does not initiate the movement it makes sure the movement is smooth and controlled. It is also the region of the brain that is largely affected if you drink too much alcohol, which will be evident by staggering and the inability to stay balanced.

Coordination is the ability to perform actions smoothly and effectively, without hesitant, jerky movements. For example, applying mascara without poking yourself in the eye or taking a sip of hot coffee and not spilling it. Good coordination allows us to perform activities such as dancing, driving, eating and playing sports. In Table 23.2 I have listed some coordination exercises and activities you can perform to help improve your eye-hand coordination as well as balance.

Flexibility Can Reduce the Risk of Injury

A muscle/tendon strain or a ligament sprain occurs when the joint has stretched to the point where it cannot go any further, resulting in an injury. Most people have tight rotator cuff (shoulder muscles) and hamstrings because we spend most of our days in the flexed position such as driving or sitting. As a result overtime our flexors (e.g. hamstring, hip flexors, and chest muscles) become tight and less flexible.

Flexibility is measured by the ability to move a joint. Flexibility can reduce injury and improve physical performance. However, too much flexibility can leave a joint feeling loose and unstable. On the other hand, having little to no flexibility will make it difficult for you to perform everyday activities such as getting dress.

I have listed a few tests in Table 23.3 that are designed to measure your joint flexibility. Perform the test and record your score in the Appendix. If you don't have a flexibility program you partake in, I encourage you to incorporate stretching and flexibility exercises into your daily routine. Yoga and Pilates are great to improve flexibility, balance, and coordination.

Flexibility Tests

Prior to performing the flexibility tests, make sure that you warm up. This will give you the best results.

Back Scratch Test: I use this test to check bilateral shoulder flexibility in patients. You will need a ruler, yardstick or measuring tape. Stand, place one hand behind your head and reach as far down your back as possible with your palms touching your back and the fingers downward. With the other hand, reach behind your back, reaching upward as far as possible, with your fingers upward and palms facing away from your body. Reaching far, attempting to touch and/or overlap the fingers. Have someone measure in inches the distance between the middle fingers (if applicable) and record. If the fingers tips are touching then the score is zero. Repeat with the opposite hand. The hand that is on the bottom is the shoulder you are testing.

Sit-and-Reach Test: Used to check hip and lower back flexibility. Sit on the floor with the bottom of your feet touching the wall. Lean forward with your arms and fingers straight and touch the wall. Have someone measure the distance between your fingertips and the wall.

Groin Flexibility Test: You will need a tape measure or a ruler. Sit on the floor with your knees bent and feet flat on the floor. Allow your knees to drop to the side as far as possible. Keeping your feet together pull your feet with your hands bringing them to your body. Measure the distance between the heels of your foot and your groin.

Thomas Test: Used to check hip and lower back flexibility. Sit on the edge of a table/bench or bed. Bend your right knee, placing your hand on the back of your thigh. Now bring the bent knee as close to your chest as possible. Record the results, then repeat on the left side.

Active Straight Leg Raise Test: Used to measure flexibility of the lower back, hamstring and calf muscles. Lay on your back with your legs straight. Lift your right leg off the table, keeping your leg straight, bring your knee toward your chest. Record the results and repeat on the left side.

You Should Know:
- You can improve your balance and coordination through weight training.
- Flexibility helps reduce your chances of an injury.
- As our bodies age, strength, balance, coordination and flexibility play a major part in maintaining our independence.
- Balance exercises can improve balance and reduce risk of falling.
- Training barefoot has it benefits such as improved joint proprioception and foot muscles strength.

Phase VII
Eating for Recovery

"Let food be your medicine and medicine be thy food."

Hippocrates

Introduction to Phase VII

What you eat is not only important in maintaining a healthy life, free from diseases and illness, but it plays a prominent role in the recovery stage. In this phase you will learn what foods you should eat and what foods you should avoid to help promote maximum healing, like those foods that promotes tissue growth and reduce inflammation.

Chapter 24

Fuel Your Nervous System

A normal functioning nervous system not only helps you go through everyday life, but it also helps you recover from diseases and illness that may afflict the body.

In my opinion, the nervous is in part the most important bodily system for this reason... it controls and regulates all other bodily systems functions which is expressed through voluntary and involuntary activities. It tells the heart how fast to beat, the lungs how wide to expand, it signals the muscle to contract and relax, and tells the stomach when to begin digestion. Therefore the entire body depends on a healthy functioning nervous system.

The nervous system has two parts: the central nervous system (CNS), which includes the brain and spinal cord and the peripheral nervous system (PNS), which includes the spinal nerves. The peripheral nervous system has the unique ability to repair and regenerate itself if it is damaged; however, once damaged to the CNS has occurred the injury is usually permanent.

For this reason, it is important to provide your nervous system with the proper nutrition that will allow it to be healthy and maintain normal function. With health conditions, such as Parkinson's and Alzheimer's affecting more than 6.3 million and 36 million worldwide, respectively, having a healthy nervous system can help prolong your days.

Like all tissues within our bodies the brain, spinal cord, and nerves all age with time. Eating foods that will help promote longevity of tissue and cells is important. In this chapter you will learn what foods you should eat to maintain a healthy nervous system which are listed in Table 24.1. What is good for the brain is also good for the heart. So whatever you eat for your brain your heart equally benefits from the same foods.

It is best to consume the vegetables and fruit in its natural form (raw) and to avoid cooking them too much, by doing so it will lose most of its nutritional value.

Note: Anti-oxidants fight by slowing the aging process of cells by preventing free radicals (which cause oxidative damage to cells).

You Should Know:
- What is good for the brain and nervous system is also good for the heart and cardiovascular system.
- Anti-oxidants are powerful in eliminating the body of free radicals, which cause oxidative damages to cells.
- The nervous system is the most important system because it controls all bodily functions, voluntary and involuntary.

Table 24.1 Foods You Should Eat to Fuel Your Nervous System

Food	Vitamins and Minerals	Benefits
Dark Green Leafy Vegetables (e.g. spinach, Swiss chard, kale, collard, turnip, mustard greens, cabbage); Lettuces (Romaine lettuce, green and red leaf lettuce, arugula, and butter head) and broccoli	• Vitamin A, C, and K • Potassium • Calcium • Folate • Iron	• Improve eyesight • Bone health • Blood clotting • Inhibit the growth of certain cancers • Enhance and maintain heart and brain function • Anti-oxidants (fight free radicals)
Whole grains	• Fiber • Vitamin B and E • Phytochemicals • Iron • Copper • Zinc • Magnesium • Carbohydrates • Protein • Healthy fats	• Lowers cholesterol. • Lowers diabetes risk. • Protection against certain cancers. • Normal bowel function. • Prevent constipation. • Reduce risk of heart disease. • Reduce risk of obesity. • Weight control. • Contain anti-oxidants.
Brown rice	• Selenium • Manganese • Fiber • Anti-oxidants	• Normal bowel function. • Weight control.
Cocoa	• Selenium • Anti-oxidant • Copper • Magnesium • Vitamins E and K	• Reduce risk of chronic illnesses such as cancer, stroke and coronary heart disease.
Nuts (e.g. walnuts almonds, cashews, Brazil nuts)	• Omega-3-fatty acids • Copper • Manganese • Molybdenum • Biotin • Vitamin E • Folate	• Reduce risk of certain cancers (e.g. prostate and breast). • Anti-inflammatory • Reduce risk of heart disease. • Weight control. • Improved reproduction in men. • Support brain health. • Lower cholesterol. • Improve heart function.

Garlic	• Manganese • Vitamin B6 and C • Fiber • Selenium • Calcium • Copper • Potassium • Phosphorus • Iron and Vitamin B1	• Boost function of immune system. • Reduce blood pressure. • Lower risk of heart disease. • Contains anti-oxidants. • Reduce risk of Alzheimer's disease and dementia. • Reduce risk of certain cancers (colon, rectal and stomach).
Olive oil	• Contain anti-oxidants	• Reduce inflammation. • Lowers total cholesterol. • Reduce risk of cardiovascular disease. • Lower blood pressure. • Weight loss and management. • Help with insulin levels and blood sugar control.
Red wine (in moderation)	• Contain anti-oxidants	• Heart health. • Raises high-density lipoprotein (HDL) cholesterol "good cholesterol." • Reduce the formation of blood clots. • Prevent artery damage.
Green tea	• Contains anti-oxidants	• Reduce growth of certain cancers (bladder, breast, lung, stomach, pancreatic, and colorectal). • Prevent clogging in arteries. • Burn fat. • Reduce risk of Alzheimer's and Parkinsons's disease. • Improve cholesterol levels.

Cold water fish (e.g. sardines, salmon, herring, mackerel, halibut, black cod and Arctic char)	• Omega-3-fatty acids • Vitamin D	• Anti-inflammatory. • Increase collagen .production • Improves bone density and strength. • Brain function. • Improved cardiovascular health. • Eye health.
Blueberries	• Anti-oxidants • Vitamin C, B complex, and E • Copper • Selenium • Zinc • Iron • Sodium • Potassium • Fiber • Manganese	• Helps lower cholesterol. • Reduce risk of cardiovascular disease and diabetes. • Anti-bacterial. • Improve immune function. • Reduce belly fat. • Brain, urinary system and eye health. • Help manage cholesterol levels. • Maintain normal bowel function. • Reduce the growth of certain cancers (e.g. colon). • Reduce risk of certain cancers (e.g. ovarian).

Chapter 25
Drink Water for Life

"Water, thou hast no taste, no color, no odor; canst not be defined, art relished while every mysterious. Not necessary to life, but rather life itself, thou fillest us with a gratification that exceeds the delight of the senses."

Antoine de Saint-Exupery

"Water flows from the high in the mountains
Water runs deep in the Earth
Miraculously, water comes to us,
And sustains all life."

Thich Nhat Hanh

Water Sustains All Life

Water is that one substance that without it, life will cease. Water is the essence of our existence and sustains our being. Water is essential. It supports and promotes life. There has been a debate as to how much water a person should consume on a daily basis, some say their body weight in ounces, and others say half their body weight and finally, the idea of 8 glasses of 8 ounces of water a day. The truth is this... there are no scientific studies that pinpoint exactly how much water we really need. We all can agree that we must consume water on a daily basis to maintain bodily function. We also know that if we consume too little we can become severely dehydrated and if we consume too much, this can create problems such as water intoxication, which is rare.

Are You Getting Enough Water?
According to the Institute of Medicine the recommendation for daily water intake can be seen in Table 25.1.

A good way to measure if you are consuming enough water is to simply check your urine. If it is a dark yellow color, then you may need to drink more water and if it is clear, then you are getting enough. We should consume as much water during the winter months as we do the rest of the year, to avoid dry skin and dehydration.

There are wonderful benefits of water, from regulating your blood pressure to providing a natural daily detoxification for the liver and kidneys. Surprisingly I have met people who don't like to drink water and the idea of drinking bottle(s) of water makes them uncomfortable. Yes, we do get water from our foods, but it will not be enough to sustain us on daily basis. I generally recommend patients to use Dixie cups to get their water. Basically, drink one to three "shots of water" from the Dixie cups (which is about three ounces), every hour on the hour while they are at work/school. By breaking up into smaller ounces, it seems less intimidating. And at the end of the work/school day, they would have consumed between twenty-four to seventy-two ounces, which is a good start.

Try adding fresh fruit or vegetables such as lemon, oranges and cucumbers to the water for extra flavor.

How to Check if You're Dehydrated
To check for dehydration, simply pinch your skin on the back of your

hand. If the skin springs back quickly, then more likely you are not de-hydrate, but if the skin lags and returns slowly chances are you need to drink water. If you feel thirsty you are probably dehydrated.

Signs of Dehydration

- Increased thirst
- Dry mouth
- Weakness
- Dizziness or lightheadedness
- Heart palpitations
- Confusion
- Sluggishness, tired or fatigue
- Inability to sweat
- Decreased urine output
- Headaches
- Nausea and vomiting
- Muscle cramps
- Loss of appetite
- Dry cough
- Dark-colored urine

If you or someone you know is dehydrated seek medical attention im-mediately.

Avoid Dehydration

- Don't wait until you feel thirsty to drink water. Sometimes hunger can be mistaken for thirst.
- Drink water at least twenty ounces prior to exercising or par-ticipating in any sporting activity.
- Drink a glass of water upon rising in the morning.
- Avoid excessive consumption of alcoholic and caffeinated bev-

erages such as coffee, tea, and soda.
- During the summer, keep water on hand.

Table 25.1 Recommended Daily Water Intake	
Men	Women
125 ounces (3.7 liters)	90 ounces (2.7 liters)

Drink Water for Healing

Whether you have recently suffered from an injury (trauma) or are dealing with a chronic condition, drinking water can help ease pain and promote healing. Water is available in abundance and should be consumed regularly to ensure that you keep your body functioning. It has many benefits from helping to maintain or lose weight to keeping your skin beautiful and healthy.

Benefits of Drinking Water
- Help to lose/maintain weight
- Healthy skin
- Fights infection
- Get rid of body toxins
- Healthy heart
- Prevent joint pains such as arthritis
- Normal bowel movements
- Prevent constipation
- Reduce risk of certain cancer
- Improves productivity
- Maintain body fluids

You Should Know
- 65 percent of our bodies are composed of water.

- Insufficient water intake can lead to urinary tract infections, digestive problems (e.g. constipation), headaches and dry skin.
- Daily water intake can help regulate blood pressure, lubricate the joints, and regulate digestion.

Chapter 26
Combat Inflammation

Inflammation is a necessary immune response; it is how the body responds to an injury or infection.

Once damage has occurred to tissues, inflammation and swelling accumulate in and around the injured area. The swelling serves a purpose tto prevent further movement of the joints which can cause more damage to the area by excessive movements and the inflammation is a result of the increase of blood flow into the area. However, prolong inflammation and swelling can be damaging to a joint. For example, arthritis is a condition that involves inflammation of one or more joint such as Gout or Rheumatoid Arthritis. A complaint of arthritis or joint inflammation is joint pain, muscle stiffness, tenderness and pain during movement of the joint(s).

Having a diet that is rich in anti-inflammatory foods can help decrease the symptoms you may experience such as pain, muscle stiffness and difficulty moving the joint. In this chapter you will learn what foods create inflammation within the body, hence the foods you should avoid if you are experiencing joint inflammation and swelling; and what foods you should intake to help reduce joint swelling and inflammation.

There are wonderful benefits of consuming foods that are anti-inflammatory, such as reducing risk of cardiovascular disease.

Anti-Inflammatory Foods: You Should Avoid if You Are Experiencing Inflammation

Inflammation is a necessary immune response; it is how the body responds to an injury and infection. However, prolong inflammation can be very damaging to the body, by damaging cells and joints. I have listed foods that are anti-inflammatory that if consumed can help relieve Symptoms of pain, see Table 26.1.

Note: These foods may reduce pain and inflammation in some patients, while it may exacerbate the symptoms in others. Not everything works for everyone. See what works best for you and do that.

Table 26.1 Anti-Inflammatory Foods

Anti-Inflammatory Foods	Other Benefits if Consumed Regularly
Foods to consume—that combat inflammation	
Dark leafy green vegetables (e.g. kale, collard, turnip, chard, spinach, mustard, bok choy, salad greens and broccoli)	• Contain vitamins A, C, K, and B complex. • Contain calcium, potassium, and folate. • Low calorie. • Low carbohydrate. • Low sodium. • Low cholesterol. • High anti-oxidants. • Reduce risk of certain cancers (e.g. stomach, breast, and skin). • Reduce risk of cardiovascular disease.
Nuts (e.g. walnuts, almonds, macadamia, hazelnuts, cashews, and pecans)	• Can lower low-density lipoprotein (LDL) or "bad" cholesterol. • Reduce risk of cardiovascular disease. • Contain healthy omega-3 fatty acids. • Fiber, which helps lower cholesterol. • Contain vitamin E.
Cold water fish (e.g. salmon, smelt, sardines, anchovies, black cod)	• Contain healthy omega-3 fatty acids.
Whole grains	• Contain dietary fiber. • Contain B-complex vitamins. • Contains iron, magnesium and selenium. • May help reduce blood cholesterol. • May lower risk of heart disease and type 2 diabetes. • Help maintain healthy bowel function. • Helps body form red blood cells. • Helps build and maintain bones and muscles. • Helps maintain a healthy immune system.

Lean protein (e.g. chicken, fish and dry beans)	• Great source for protein, which are the building blocks for body tissue (e.g. bones and muscle). • Contain B-vitamin complex and vitamin E. • Contains iron, zinc, and magnesium.
Spices (e.g. ginger and curry)	• Help fight against colds.
Peppers*	• Anti-oxidants (fight free radicals).
Tomatoes	• Contain vitamins A, C, K, and B-complex. • Contains folate, potassium, magnesium, phosphorus and copper. • Low sodium. • Low cholesterol. • Low calorie. • Protect the eyes and skin. • Build and strengthen bones. • Reduce risk of certain cancers (e.g. prostate, cervical, mouth, throat, prostate, and ovarian). • Anti-oxidants (fight free radicals). • Help regulate blood sugar.
Beets	• Low calorie. • Anti-oxidant.
Herbs (e.g. garlic)	• Anti-bacterial. • Anti-fungal. • Can be used to treat fevers, headaches, upset stomachs, congestion, bronchitis, asthma, high cholesterol and atherosclerosis. • Helps lower blood pressure. • Helps lower blood sugar. • Used to prevent certain cancers (e.g. breast, stomach, prostate, and lung). • Help reduce the risk of cardiovascular disease.
Onion	• Contains vitamin C and A. • Help regulate blood sugar. • Reduce risk of cardiovascular disease.

Olive oil	• Help lower cholesterol. • Contains anti-oxidants. • Help lower blood pressure. • Improve bone strength.
Berries	• Contain anti-oxidants and vitamin C. • Contains folate and fiber.
Tart cherries	• Reduce pain and inflammation.

Pro-Inflammatory Foods: Foods that Promote Inflammation

These are foods that should be avoided if you suffer from arthritis or any other inflammatory condition such as Alzheimer's. See Table 26.2 for a list of foods that create an immune response within the body that is expressed as inflammation, in addition to other reasons why you should limit or avoid consuming these products.

Table 26.2 Pro-Inflammatory Foods	
Pro-Inflammatory Foods	**Reasons Why You Should Limit or Avoid Consuming**
Foods to avoid—that promote inflammation	
Foods high in sugar	• Foods high in sugar are usually processed such as pastries, sodas and candy bars) which contain no vitamins and no minerals, hence empty calories. • Can create insulin resistance. • Deposition of fat in the liver • Risk of becoming overweight. • Increase risk of diabetes and heart disease.
Foods high in saturated fat	• Increase risk of heart disease. • Increase cholesterol. • Increase risk of heart attack and/or stroke. • Increase LDL "bad" cholesterol levels.
Cooking oils (e.g. cottonseed, safflower, corn and sunflower)	• High in saturated fat. • May contain natural toxins. • Increase risk of cardiovascular disease such as cancer and diabetes.
Foods containing trans-fats (e.g. deep fried foods and fast foods)	• Increase risk of cardiovascular disease, diabetes, cancer and obesity.
Milk and dairy products	• Acid forming product. • May contain hormones and antibiotics.
Red meat	• Increase risk of heart disease. • High in saturated fat.
Processed meat (e.g. sausage, luncheon meats)	• Contain nitrates, when consumed in large quantities can increase risk of cancer. • When consumed in large quantities can increase risk of death by 44%.
Refined grains	• Increase accumulation of abdominal fat. • Increase risk of atherosclerosis. • Increase risk of diabetes.

Artificial food additives (e.g. monosodium glutamate, MSG)	• Some individuals who have consumed too much MSG have experience headache, numbness and tingling. • Food coloring maybe linked to hyperactivity in children. • Food preservatives may trigger asthmatic symptoms and migraines in people with sensitivity.
Whatever foods you are sensitive too (e.g. gluten-products for some people)	

Whenever you consume a food that you are sensitive too, your body has an inflammatory immune response, whether the response is expressed through pain, discomfort, bloating, gas or diarrhea. Those foods should be avoided.

You Should Know:
- Inflammation is a natural immune response to infection and injury.
- Consuming a diet that is anti-inflammatory can help improve your overall health.
- Prolonged inflammatory conditions (such as arthritis) can be damaging not only to the joints but also to the other bodily parts.

Chapter 27

Boost Tissue Repair

"Healing is a matter of time, but it is sometimes also a matter of opportunity."

Hippocrates

Whenever your body suffers from an injury or trauma, there will always be some form of tissue damage whether it is great or small. In addition to exercising, eating foods that will promote tissue repair will be to your benefit. Body tissues are comprised of a group of cells that work together to perform a specific function.

In this chapter you will learn what foods you can consume that will aid in the growth and repair of damaged tissue of the muscles and bones. Foods rich in calcium, folic acid, magnesium, phosphorus and vitamin D are important in repairing, maintaining and strengthening the musculoskeletal system.

Calcium and Vitamin D

Calcium
Calcium is the most abundant mineral in the human body. It plays an important role in muscle contraction as well as the growth and devel-

opment of bone. However in order for calcium to be absorbed into the tissues, vitamin D must be present. Calcium is one of the most important minerals of the body and having a deficiency of calcium can lead to weaken fragile bones. An increased in calcium concentration in our blood is an indication of healing. Table 27.1 lists foods rich in calcium.

Table 27.1 Foods Rich in Calcium
Dark Green Leafy Vegetables (kale, mustard greens, turnip, arugula, and collards), low fat cheese (e.g. mozzarella, reduced fat Swiss, parmesan, and cottage cheese), low fat milk and yogurt, Chinese cabbage (pak choi, bok choy), fortified soy products (e.g. tofu), okra, broccoli and spinach, green snap beans, nuts (e.g. walnuts), and fish (e.g. sardines, pink salmon, anchovies, and shrimp).

Vitamin D

Vitamin D is produced naturally in the skin when it is exposed to the sun. In order to get enough vitamin D by sun exposure, people who are already tan need to spend at least fifteen to twenty minutes a day in the sun. More time should be spent in the sun for people who have darker skin and less time for people with very light or pale skin, in order for the skin to absorb the UV rays. It is important in absorbing calcium and maintaining normal blood levels of bone minerals, calcium and phosphorus. You can also get daily Vitamin D by eating fresh fish. See Table 27.2 for a list of foods rich in Vitamin D.

Table 27.2 Foods Rich in Vitamin D
Fish (e.g. tuna, mackerel, and salmon), beef liver, cheese, egg yolks, and fortified foods that contain vitamin D, such as dairy products, juice and cereals.

Folic Acid (also known as Vitamin B9, Folacin and Folate)

Most of us know how important it is for a pregnant woman to get the recommended daily intake of folic acid (folate) to prevent birth deficits in the baby. Folic acid plays an important role in tissue maintenance and repair. In fact, it determines the rate at which tissues are repaired.

Table 27.3 Foods Rich in Folic Acid (Folate)
Green leafy vegetables (spinach, collard greens, turnip greens, mustard greens, and romaine lettuces), fruits (especially citrus fruits), beans, peas, and lentils, enriched breads, cereals, and other grain products, asparagus, broccoli, cauliflower, and spinach, avocado, okra, Brussels sprouts, nuts (e.g. almonds and peanuts), and seeds (e.g. flax and sunflower), beets, corn, celery, carrots and squash.

Magnesium

Magnesium has many functions within the body such as nerve, muscle and bone health. It helps form connective tissue, repair damaged tissue and is often used to treat many conditions, such as chest pain, high blood pressure, osteoporosis, fibromyalgia and to prevent constipation by regulating bowel movements. Table 27.4 lists foods that are rich in magnesium.

Table 27.4 Foods Rich in Magnesium
Dark Green Leafy Vegetables (e.g. spinach, Swiss chard, and kale), nuts (e.g. almonds, brazil, cashews, pine nuts, mixed nuts, peanuts and walnuts), seeds (e.g. sesame and pumpkin), fish (e.g. mackerel, Pollock, turbot, and tuna), beans and lentils (e.g. white beans, French beans, black-eyed peas, kidney beans, chickpeas, garbanzo, and pinto beans), whole grains, avocado, low-fat dairy products, and fruits (e.g. bananas).

Phosphorus

Like calcium, Phosphorus it is essential for bone health, however, it also plays an important role in the growth, repair and maintenance of all cells and tissues. It is the second most abundant mineral in the human body. Table 27.5 lists foods that are rich in phosphorus.

Table 27.5 Foods Rich in Phosphorus
Seeds (e.g. pumpkin, sunflower, chia, sesame, and flaxseeds), cheese, fish (e.g. salmon, whitefish, cod, tuna and mackerel), shellfish, nuts (e.g. almonds, cashews, pistachio and pine nuts), pork (sirloin cut), lean beef, low fat dairy products, tofu, lentils and beans.

You Should Know:

- Eating a variety of fresh fruits, vegetables and lean meats will help with the growth and development of all tissues and increase your energy level.
- Most vegetables and fruits contain all the daily nutrients you need.
- Dark green leafy vegetables contain essential vitamins and minerals, such as calcium, vitamin D, phosphorus and magnesium.
- You do not have to consume dairy products to be healthy. There are plenty of foods such as dark green leafy vegetables that contain sufficient amounts of calcium than milk.

Phase VIII

You Deserve a Pain-Free Life

"Find a place inside where there's joy, and the joy will burn out the pain."

Joseph Campbell

"Pain is temporary. It may last a minute, or an hour, or a day, or a year, but eventually it will subside and something else will take its place. If I quit, however, it lasts forever."

Lance Armstrong

Introduction to Phase VIII

We all know someone who may suffer from a chronic condition that evokes a type of pain, such as physical, emotion or mental. We are all deserving of a pain-free life. A life that is full of joy, peace, and harmony. Although pain is necessary as it teaches us those things to avoid that can be potentially harmful to us; however, constant pain isn't normal. It prevents you from living a life in happiness and abundance. In this phase you will learn how you can begin to live a life pain-free. Whether you suffer from physical, mental or emotional pain, the information contained herein can be useful to you.

Chapter 28
The Body Does What the Mind Tells It to Do

*"The art of healing comes from nature, not from the physician.
Therefore the physician must start from nature, with an open mind."*
Paracelsus

*"Ill-health of body or of mind, is defeat. Health alone is victory.
Let all men, if they can manage it contrive to be healthy!"*
Thomas Carlyle

Healing Begins in the Mind
Every thought, every action, and every feeling/emotion begins in the mind. To be healed, we must first think about healing. There is a term in the medical field called hypochondriac, in whom a person perceives (thinks) they have a medical condition, but in reality they don't. Your mind can make you sick and your mind can also heal you. The power is up to you. Sickness and health is a state of the mind and our bodies merely reflect the state. If you are faced with a bodily affliction consider thinking I am healed. Consider how good it feels to be healthy, joyful and happy. Consider how wonderful it is to be able to do the things you love. A wonderful thing happens when you begin to change your perception.

Smile. You have a lot to be thankful for. The simple act of smiling or exercising, releases hormones called endorphins within the brain that has many functions such as reducing our perception of pain and enhancing our immune response. So, not only does smiling make you appear friendly, receptive and pleasant, it makes you feel better. You can't be both miserable and smiling at the same time. It just doesn't work that way.

What You Think You Are... You Are

What you think you are, you essentially are or will become. If you think you will always have chronic pain, diseases and sickness then you will always have it. The majority of people, when faced with a trauma, think the worse. Most people are reactive rather that proactive. They wait until something happens before they take action or make a change. Why not take action and initiate positive change? What do you have to lose?

Get Rid of "Stinking Thinking"

Negative thoughts attract negative behavior and undesired outcomes. Your poor thoughts expressed through your poor choices (actions/behavior) will lead to your poor lifestyle. How you view yourself has a lot to do with how you treat yourself and others. As a man thinketh so is he. My question to you is: What are you thinking? Do you think you will not be healed? Do you think you will have this condition, illness or disease for the rest of your life? Do you think no one can help you? Do you think you are hopeless? Negative thoughts like these will not help your situation or help your healing, it will only worsen your symptoms, weaken your faith and leave you hopeless.

Your Thoughts Can Heal You

What you think can either build you up or tear you down. Thoughts are not invisible flashes that come into our minds. Thoughts are things.

Our thoughts can bring us life or bring us to the doorstep of death. Our thoughts can bring us peace, joy, happiness, health, and life. Therefore, we must think with intention. Think with a definite purpose in mind. The majority of people do not put any thought into thinking. They allow others to do the thinking for them. Not all of the thoughts we think are our own. Thoughts from our friends, family, television, radio, the Internet, movies, etc. will have an influence on us one way or the other. Although we do not have complete control of thoughts, we do have complete control on whether these thoughts are displayed through our actions/behavior. We decide what thoughts we want to become reality, to be manifested in our lives. Nevertheless, we are a sum of our thoughts. That is why we must begin to think deliberately and with a purpose because external forces at times persuade our thoughts. So, again, what are you thinking?

Connect with Your Source of Healing

You have the power within you, within your mind to heal yourself. Thinking positively about your situation can lead to a positive outcome. What we think is expressed by our speech and deeds. If you think you are healed you will begin to speak and behave/act as someone who is healed.

We are born with all of the tools to be self-healing and self-maintaining. We must learn to tap into our inner source, to our inner power, to give rise to the power that lies dormant within us. Replace those negative thoughts with positive thoughts. Begin to replace negative, self-defeating thoughts with positive, life-enhancing thoughts. Thinking positive is necessary for boosting and maintaining your health.

You Should Know:
- Think positively and with intention.
- You have the power to heal yourself and the power lies within you.

- We are (and/or become) what we think about.
- Your healing begins in your mind.

Chapter 29
Affirming Your Health

"The greatest wealth is health."

Virgil

"Health is a state of complete physical, mental and social well-being, and not merely the absence of disease or infirmity."
World Health Organization, WHO, 1948

You Deserve a Pain-Free Life

Know that you deserve a life free of pain, full of joy peace and happiness. You deserve it. It is your birthright. Regardless of your current circumstances or where you are presently in life, you can change your outcome by changing your attitude. Pain is merely a perception; it is what our brains interpret to be potentially harmful or dangerous to us. This is why we tend to avoid pain, whether it is physical, emotion or mental. Our perception is our reality; it is how we see the world. Change your perception change your reality.

Affirmations are powerful positive statements, that when repeated daily, frequently and with faith can transform your life. All that you need and want from life resides within you. You have the power to change, the power to create a better life and to create the life you want to live.

Remember, the body does what the mind tells it to do. There is a powerful connection between the mind and body. Believe and ye shall receive. Tap into this connection and start healing.

Affirming Your Health

I have listed a few health affirmations. When you start to use them; your life will began to change. Make it personal by creating your own personalized affirmations. Find a place that is quiet. Say them out-loud, with authority and with full faith believing in the words that you are affirming.

- I am healthy, whole and complete.
- Every cell of my body is healthy.
- Every day in every way I am becoming healthier and healthier.
- I am strong, healthy and full of energy.
- Being healthy is my birthright.
- I have the power to heal myself.
- I am already healed.
- I am healed from all non-life threatening and life-threatening conditions.
- I am free of muscle and joint pain.
- My muscles and joints are healthy.
- I am thankful for my healthy body and my mind.
- I love myself and I am perfectly healthy.
- I feed my body healthy nutritious foods.
- I get regular exercise because it makes me feel good and healthy.
- My physical body is perfectly healthy.
- I am ready to enjoy a life full of health, peace and happiness.
- I only attract healthy things into my life.

Express Gratitude and Being Thankful

"Feeling gratitude and not expressing it is like wrapping a present and not giving it."

William Arthur Ward

When the going gets tough and the road gets lonely, it seems hard to keep a positive attitude. Know that you are never alone. There are people who love and care for you. Despite hard-times knowing that trouble don't last always give us hope. Look for happiness in your troubled times. Happiness is not found externally, but it is found inside of you. Waking up in the morning with the sunlight shining through the windows and hearing the birds' sing is enough to bring a smile to your face. Realizing that you still have function of your eyes and ears. Expressing gratitude and giving thanks for the things you do have. Too many people focus on what they don't have and not on what they do have. I am guilty of this as well. However, once I learned the power of positive thinking and expressing gratitude and thanks for the things I do have, my life began to change for the better.

The truth of the matter is we create our own happiness. We create our own world experience. Seek the good in all things, even in situations that are deemed unfortunate. If you want to change your world, change your perception. There are many ways to express gratitude. It begins with the feeling of being thankful. Those who express daily gratitude are often happier, more sympathetic, and forgiving.

You Should Know:
- You deserve a pain-free life.
- Begin to start living a pain-free life today. Affirm it.
- Profess your healing, receive your healing and accept your healing.

- Be thankful and express gratitude for your healthy life.
- Express daily appreciation for your life and health.
- Be thankful for what you DO have. Don't focus on what you don't have.

Phase IX
Making the Change

"Everyone thinks of changing the world, but no one thinks of changing himself."

Leo Tolstoy

Introduction to Phase IX

Most of us want to make a difference in the world. To make it a better place for our generation and the generations to come. Whether it is through monetary contributions or volunteering we believe that our efforts, if used in a positive way, will evoke change. There is no doubt in my mind that you can create change. However, we must first consider our own lives before we can consider someone else. Are you being the loving, kind and generous person to yourself? Are we feeding ourselves nutritious food, getting enough rest, and exercising regularly? How are you treating your body? How are you treating you?

If you are unhappy with your current health status, by simply making up your mind that you want to change, is the first step towards living a healthy lifestyle. There are a few steps to follow that I will discuss later. First, think you can change, believe you can change, know you can change and then put forth the work that is required to change.

In this phase you will learn the necessary steps on how to improve your life. The information will mean nothing to you unless you put it to practical use. Learn the information, share it with your friends and family and visit it often. The more you know, the more resourceful and useful you can be to yourself and someone else.

Chapter 30

Implementation of the Plan

"Unless you are prepared to give up something valuable you will never be able to truly change at all, because you'll be forever in the control of things you can't give up."

Andy Law

You've Decided to Change, Now What?

It is not easy to change. Most people do not change but will remain the same their entire lives wishing and hoping that they did things differently. When you decide to change you must take the necessary steps to move forward. In this chapter I have outlined six steps to take to begin living a healthy lifestyle.

Step One: Decide You Want to Change

No one can change you but you. If you are unhappy with your current lifestyle, do something about it. Write down the reasons why you want to change, the pros (benefits and rewards) and cons (punishments) for changing. Once you make up your mind that you want to change, it's time to do some work.

Step Two: Write Down Your Goals

Write down your goals. A goal must be measurable, reachable and realistic with a deadline (due date). By writing down your goals, you are making an agreement with yourself. You are holding yourself accountable for your thoughts and actions from this point forward. *"Successful people are successful because they know where they are going." Earl Nightingale.*

An example of a health goal is: I want to reduce my cholesterol by ten points by December 31, 2018.

Step Three: Have Faith and Believe You Can Change

Believing is half the battle. Believe that you can change and you will. Disregard past situations in which you attempted to implement change, but it did not work out in your favor. This time will be different. The past is the past. Live in the present moment, in the now. What you do now will help shape and mold your immediate and distant future.

Step Four: Get to Work

You must do work. Nothing will happen unless you take action. Believing you can change, by performing the necessary works it takes to change. It is not enough to simply believe you must work at your belief. Faith without works is dead. You have the faith, now you must prove your faith through your actions (deeds and speech). Creating an action plan will be helpful in pursuing your goals.

For example, I will reduce my cholesterol by ten points by December 31, 2018. I will do so by exercising at least three times a week, drinking one hundred ounces of water daily, and eating at least thirty-five grams of fiber a day.

Step Five: Witness the Change

Pay attention and begin to notice how things start to change around you, such as your attitude or circumstances. Are things improving for the better for you? Do you feel more energetic, happier, and alive? Do people start to notice the change in you? If so, keep doing what you're doing and keep pressing forward. Stay focus and keep your eyes on the prize. You're on the right path! If something is not working out, try something else. Don't give up and never settle for less, always aim for the best.

Step Six: Testify

Share your journey with someone. It doesn't matter if you are just getting starting or if you are in the middle, sharing your story will not only encourage you and keep you motivated, but you may just encourage someone else to change. Enjoy the journey and remember it is a slow, steady process. Remember to express gratitude and thanks for what you do have.

You Should Know:

- Change requires action, so get to work.
- Healthy living is a lifestyle, not a phase.
- Write down your goals and take the necessary action steps to acquire your goals.
- Believe in yourself and know that you can change.
- Share your journey with someone else.
- Change doesn't occur overnight, it is a process.
- Remember, you deserve to live a healthy life free of disease.

Closing Remarks

Congratulations! You have completed this book. Hopefully the information written was useful and helpful to you. Unfortunately reading this book is not enough, you must put what you have learned to action. Then and only then, you will start to change, improve and see remarkable results. Most of us know someone who suffers from chronic pain who could probably benefit from the information written in this book. Share the information with your friends, family and co-workers.

Appendix

Table 22.1 Strength and Endurance Tests	
Test	Your Score
Pull-up or Chin-up	
Push-up	
Flexed Arm Hang *(for women or youth)*	
One Minute Sit-up	
Back Extension	
Low Plank	
Dead-Man Sit-Up	
Squat	

Table 22.2 Pull-up or Chin-up		
Score	Men	Women
Excellent	20+	10+
Good	13-19	5-9
Above Average	11-13	2-4
Average	8-10	1
Below Average	4-7	0-1
Poor	1-3	0
Very Poor	0	0

Table 22.3 Push-ups (Men)						
Age	17-19	20-29	30-39	40-49	50-59	60-65
Excellent	>56	>47	>41	>34	>31	>30
Good	47-56	39-47	34-41	28-34	25-31	24-30
Above Average	35-46	30-39	25-33	21-28	18-24	17-30
Average	19-34	17-29	13-24	11-20	9-17	6-16
Below Average	11-18	10-16	8-12	6-10	5-8	3-5
Poor	4-10	4-9	2-7	1-5	1-4	1-2
Very Poor	<4	<4	<2	0	0	0

Above information taken from the book The Y's Way to Physical Fitness, 3rd Edition.

Table 22.3 Push-ups (Women)						
Age	17-19	20-29	30-39	40-49	50-59	60-65
Excellent	>35	>36	>37	>31	>25	>23
Good	28-35	30-36	31-37	25-31	21-25	19-23
Above Average	21-27	23-29	22-30	18-24	15-20	13-18
Average	11-20	12-22	10-21	8-17	7-14	5-12
Below Average	6-10	7-11	5-9	4-7	3-6	2-4
Poor	2-5	2-6	1-4	1-3	1-2	1
Very Poor	0-1	0-1	0	0	0	0

Above information taken from the book The Y's Way to Physical Fitness, 3rd Edition.

Table 22.4 Flexed Arm Hang

	Men	Women
Excellent	90+ seconds	60+ seconds
Good	60-90 seconds	31-59 seconds
Above Average	31-59 seconds	16-30 seconds
Average	30 seconds	15 seconds
Below Average	21-29 seconds	8-14 seconds
Poor	10-20 seconds	1-7 seconds
Very Poor	0-10 seconds	0 seconds

Table 22.5 One-Minute Sit Up Test (Men)

Age	18-25	26-35	36-45	46-55	56-65	65+
Excellent	>49	>45	>41	>35	>31	>28
Good	44-49	40-45	35-41	29-35	25-31	22-28
Above Average	39-43	35-39	30-34	25-28	21-24	19-21
Average	35-38	31-34	27-29	22-24	17-20	15-18
Below Average	31-34	29-30	23-26	18-21	13-16	11-14
Poor	25-30	22-28	17-22	13-17	9-12	7-10
Very Poor	<25	<22	<17	<13	<9	<7

Above information taken from the book The Y's Way to Physical Fitness, 3rd Edition.

Table 22.5 One-Minute Sit Up Test (Women)						
Age	18-25	26-35	36-45	46-55	56-65	65+
Excellent	>43	>39	>33	>27	>24	>23
Good	37-43	33-39	27-33	22-27	18-24	17-23
Above Average	33-36	29-32	23-26	18-21	13-17	14-16
Average	29-32	25-28	19-22	14-17	10-12	11-13
Below Average	25-28	21-24	15-18	10-13	7-9	5-10
Poor	18-24	13-20	7-14	5-9	3-6	2-4
Very Poor	<18	<13	<7	<5	<3	<2

Above information taken from the book The Y's Way to Physical Fitness, 3rd Edition.

Table 22.6 Back Extension Text		
	Men	Women
Excellent	150+ seconds	150+ seconds
Good	75-150 seconds	75-150 seconds
Above Average	46-74 seconds	46-74 seconds
Average	30-45 seconds	30-45 seconds
Below Average	21-30 seconds	21-30 seconds
Poor	11-20 seconds	11-20 seconds
Very Poor	0-10 seconds	0-10 seconds

Table 22.7 Low Plank Text		
	Men	Women
Excellent	150+ seconds	150+ seconds
Good	75-150 seconds	75-150 seconds
Above Average	46-74 seconds	46-74 seconds
Average	30-45 seconds	30-45 seconds
Below Average	21-30 seconds	21-30 seconds
Poor	11-20 seconds	11-20 seconds
Very Poor	0-10 seconds	0-10 seconds

Table 12.8 Dead-Man Sit-Up (Men and Women)	
Pass	Fail
Sit completely up without using hands, bending the knees and the legs do not lift off the floor.	• Unable to sit-up • Knees bend • Legs lift off the floor • Use arms

Table 22.9 Squat Test (Men)					
Age	20-29	30-39	40-49	50-59	60+
Excellent	>34	>32	>29	>26	>23
Good	33-34	30-32	27-29	24-26	21-23
Above Average	30-32	27-29	24-26	21-23	18-20
Average	27-29	24-26	21-23	18-20	15-17
Below Average	24-26	21-23	18-20	15-17	12-14
Poor	21-23	18-20	15-17	12-14	9-11
Very Poor	<21	<18	<15	<12	<9

Squat Test Information taken from the e-book Total Fitness by Vince Antonetti

Table 22.9 Squat Test (Women)					
Age	20-29	30-39	40-49	50-59	60+
Excellent	>29	>26	>23	>20	>17
Good	27-29	24-26	21-23	18-20	15-17
Above Average	24-26	21-23	18-20	15-17	12-14
Average	21-23	18-20	15-17	12-14	9-11
Below Average	18-20	15-17	12-14	9-11	6-8
Poor	15-17	12-14	9-11	6-8	3-5
Very Poor	<15	<12	<9	<6	<3

Squat Test Information taken from the e-book Total Fitness by Vince Antonetti

Flexibility Test	
Test	Your Score
Sit-and-Reach	
Groin Flexibility	
Back Scratch	
Thomas	
Active Straight Leg	

Sit-and-Reach		
Score	Men	Women
Excellent	Palms on wall	Palms on wall
Good	Fingers touch	Fingers touch
Average	1/12 cm. away	1/10 cm. away
Poor	>13 cm. away	>11 cm. away

http://www.netfit.co.uk/fitness/test/flexibility-test.htm

Groin Flexibility Test	
Ratings	**Score**
Excellent	5 cm.
Very Good	10 cm.
Good	15 cm.
Fair	20 cm.
Poor	25 cm. or fewer

http://www.topendsports.com/testing/tests/groin-flexibility.htm

Back Scratch Test	
Score	**Results**
Excellent	Fingers overlap
Good	Fingers touch
Average	Fingers are less than 2" apart
Poor	Fingers are more than 2" apart

Thomas Test		
Score	**Results**	**Indications**
Good	Lower leg is at a 90-degree angle or touches the floor	Good hip flexibility
Poor	Lower leg off the table/bench	Indicates tight hip flexors (particular iliopsoas)
Poor	Knee of lower leg is extended	Indicates tight hip flexors (mainly the rectus femoris)
Poor	Lower leg off the table/bench and knee is extended	Indicates tight hip flexors

Note: if lower leg extends outward this is indicative of a tight IT band.

Active Straight Leg Test		
Score	Results	Indications
Excellent	Leg remains straight and no pain in the leg	Good lower back, hamstring and calf muscle flexibility
Average	Leg remains straight but pain in the leg	Good lower back flexibility and possibly tightness of hamstring or calf muscle, depending on location of pain.
Below Average	Knee starts to straighten at or about 90 degrees	Indicates tight hamstrings or calf muscles
Poor	Knee bend before 90 degrees and/or pain in the leg	Indicates tight hamstrings and calf muscles

References

Chapter 1

Milz, S. (2012). Spine function: a concert of many different players. *Journal of Anatomy*, 221:6, 479-635. DOI: 10.1111/joa.12010

Vleeming, A. et al. (2012). The sacroiliac joint: an overview of its anatomy, function and potential clinical implications. *Journal of Anatomy, 221*(6), 537-567. DOI: 10.1111/j.1469-7580.2012.01564.x

Chapter 2

Campbell, P., Foster, N.E., Thomas, E., and Dunn, K.M. 2010). Prognostic Indicators of Low Back Pain in Primary Care: Five-Year Prospective Study. *The Journal of Pain, 11*(11), 1230-1239.

Bunn, W.B. et al. (2001). Health, safety, and productivity in a manufacturing environment. *Journal of Occupational and Environmental Medicine 43*(3), 47-55.

Smith, M.W. et al. (2001). Effect of state workplace safety laws on occupational injury rates. *Journal of Occupational and Environmental Medicine, 43*(12), 1001-1010.

Dworkn, R.H. (1997). Which individuals with acute pain are more likely to develop a chronic pain syndrome? *The Journal of Pain, 6*(2), 127-136.

Green, C.R., Wheeler, J.R., and LaPorte, F. (2003). Clinical decision making in pain management: Contributions of physicians and patient characteristics to variations in practice. *The Journal of Pain*, 4(1), 29-39.

Rosenkranz, R.R., Duncan, M.J., Rosenkranz, S.K. and Kotlt, G.S. (2013). Active lifestyles related to excellent self-rated health and quality of life: cross sectional findings from 194, 545 participants in The 45 and Up Study. *BMS Public Health*, 13(1071). Doi:10.1/186/1471-2458-13-1071.

Chapter 3

Van Den Bekerom, M.P. et al. (2012). What Is The Evidence for Rest, Ice, Compression, and Elevation Therapy in the Treatment of Ankle Sprains in Adults? *J Athl Train*, 47(4): 435-443.

Chapter 4

Nyiendo, J. et al. (2001). A descriptive study of medical and chiropractic patients with chronic low back pain and sciatica: Management by physicians (practice activities) and patients (self-management). *JMPT*, 24(9), 543-551.

Author not listed. (2014 January). *Drug Facts: Nationwide Trends*. Retrieved from www.drugabuse.gov/publications/drugfacts/nationwide-trends

Author not listed. (2011 January). *Painkillers fuel growth in drug addiction*. Retrieved from http://www.health.harvard.edu/newsletters/Harvard_Mental_Health_Letter/2011/January/painkillers-fuel-growth-in-drug-addiction

Chapter 5

Chanda, M.L., et al. (2011). Pain Characteristics Differences Between Subacute and Chronic Back Pain. *The Journal of Pain*,

12(7), 792-800.

Kindler, L.L., Jones, K.D., Perrin, N., and Bennett, R.M. (2010). Risks Factors Predicting the Development of Widespread Pain From Chronic Back or Neck Pain. *The Journal of Pain*, *11*(12): 1320-1328.

Johannes, C.B., Kim Le., T., Zhou, X., Johnston, J.A., and Dworkin, R.H. (2010). The Prevalence of Chronic Pain in United States Adults: Results of an Internet-Based Survey. *The Journal of Pain*, *11*(11): 1230-1239.

Chapter 6
No references listed.

Chapter 7

Enoch, S. (2006). Recent advances and emerging treatments. *BMJ*, *332*(7547), 962-965.

Guo, S. and DiPietro, L.A. (2010). Factors Affecting Wound Healing. *J Dent Res*, *(89)*3, 219-229.

Chapter 8
No references listed.

Chapter 9

McCarberg, B.H. (2010). Acute back pain: benefits and risks of current treatments. *Curr Med Res Opin*, *26*(1): 179-190.

Duarte, M.A. (2001). Low back pain: mechanism, diagnosis, and treatment. *JMPT*, *24*(2), 147-148.

Bialosky, J.E., et al. (2013). Spinal Manipulative Therapy- Specific Changes in Pain Sensitivity in Individuals with Low Back Pain (NCT01168999). *The Journal of Pain*, *15*(2), 136-148.

Vernon, H. (2000). Spinal manipulation for chronic low back pain: A review of evidence. *JMPT 23*(3), 224.

Bronfort, G. et al. (2001). Efficacy of spinal manipulation for chronic headache: A systematic review. *JMPT 24*(7), 457-466.

Vernon, H., Humphreys, K., and Hagino, C. (2007). Chronic Mechanical Neck Pain in Adults Treated by Manual Therapy: A Systematic Review of Change Scores in Randomized Clinical Trials. *JMPT (30)*3, 215-227.

Ferrreira, M.L, Ferreira, P.H, Latimer, J., Herbert, R. and Maher, C.G. (2009). Efficacy of spinal manipulative therapy for lower back pain of less than three months duration. *JMPT 26*(9), 593-601.

Glaser, J.A., Baltz, M.A., Nietert, P.J., and Bensen, C.V. (2001). Electrical muscle stimulation as an adjunct to exercise therapy in the treatment of nonacute low back pain: A randomized trial. *The Journal of Pain 2*(5), 295-300.

Baker, Yesmin. et al. (2014). Short Term Effects of Classic Massage Compared to Connective Tissue Massage on Pressure Pain Threshold and Muscle Relaxation Response in Women With Chronic Neck Pain: A Preliminary Study. *JMPT 37*(6), 415-421.

Shaheed, C., Maher, C.G., Williams, K.A., and McLachlan, A.J. (2014). Interventions available over the counter and advice for acute low back pain: systematic review and meta-analysis. *Pain* (15):2-15.

Kornelsen, J. et al. (2013). Default Mode Network Functional Connectivity Altered in Failed Back Surgery Syndrome. *The Journal of Pain* (14):5, 483-491.

Avellanal, M., Diaz-Raganon, G., Orts, A., and Soto, S. (2014). One-year results of an algorithmic approach for managing failed back surgery syndrome. *Pain Res Manag*

Omidi-Kashani, F., Hasankhani, E.G., and Ashjazadeh, A. (2014). Lumbar spinal stenosis: who should be fused? *Asian Spine J (8)*4, 521-530.

Watters, W.C. et al. (2014). Guideline update for the performance of fusion procedures for degenerative disease of the lumbar spine. Part 13: injection therapies, low-back pain, and lumbar fusion. *J Neurosurg Spine* 21(1): 79-90.

No author listed. (2013). What you need to know about: back pain injections. *Harv Health Lett.* 38(9):7.

Kennedy, D.J., Baker, R.M., and Rathmell, J.P. (2013). Use of spinal injections for low back pain. *JAMA* 310(16), 1736.

Chapter 10 through Chapter 13

Descarreaux, M., Normand, M.C., Laurencelle, L., and Dugas, C. (2002). Evaluation of specific home exercise program for low back pain. *JMPT (25)*8, 497-503.

Slade, S.C. and Keating, J.L. (2006). Trunk-Strengthening Exercises for Chronic Low Back Pain: A Systematic Review. *JMPT (29)*2, 163-173.

França, F.R., Burke, T.N., Caffaro, R.R., Ramos, L.A., and Marques, A.P. (2012). Effects of Muscular Stretching and Segmental Stabilization on Functional Disability and Pain in Patients with Chronic Low Back Pain: A Randomized, Controlled Trial. *JMPT 35(*4), 279-285.

Aluko, A., DeSouza, L., and Peacock, J. (2013). The Effect of Core Stability Exercises on Variations in Acceleration of Trunk Movement, Pain, and Disability During an Episode of Acute Nonspecific Low Back Pain: A Pilot Clinical Trial. JMPT *36(8), 497 504.*

Pesco, M.S., Chosa, E., and Tajima, N. (2007). Comparative Study of Hands-On Therapy With Active Exercises vs Education

With Active Exercises for the Management of Upper Back Pain. *JMPT 29(3)*, 228-235.

Bruno, P.J. (2014). The use of "stabilization exercises" to affect neuromuscular control of the lumbopelvic region: a narrative review. *Can Chiropr Assoc 58(2)*, 119-130.

Jackson J.A., Banerjee-Guénette, P., Gregory D.E., and Callaghan J.P. (2013). Should we be more on the ball? The efficacy of the accommodation training on the lumbar spine posture, muscle activity, and perceived discomfort during stability ball sitting. *Hum Factors 55(6)*, 1064-179.

Brumitt, J., Mathewson, J.W., and Meira, E.P. (2013). Core stabilization prescription, part 2: a systematic review of motor control and general (global) exercise rehabilitation approaches for patients with low back pain. *Sports Health 5(6)*, 510-513.

Chapter 14

National Research Council (US) Steering Committee for the Workshop on Work-Related Musculoskeletal Injuries: The Research Base. Washington (DC). (1999). Work-Related Musculoskeletal Disorders: Reports, Workshop Summary, and Workshop Papers *National Academies Press* (US).

Kang, D. et al. Prevention of work-related musculoskeletal disorders. *Ann Occup Environ Med (26)14*.

Halim, I. et al. Development of decision support system for analysis and solutions of prolonged standing in the workplace. *Saf Health Work (5)2*, 97-105.

Chapter 15

Rowland, G. (2004). Occupational low back pain: The critical role of functional goal setting. *The Journal of Pain (3)2*,101-106.

Arezes, P.M., Dinis-Carvalho, J., and Alves, A.C. (2014). Workplace ergonomics in lean production environments: A literature review. *Work*

Radjiyev, A., Qui, H., Xiong, S., and Nam, K. (2014). Ergonomics and sustainable development in the past two decades (1992-2011): Research trends and how ergonomics can contribute to sustainable development. *Appl Ergon*

Dropkin, J. et al. (2014). Effect of an office ergonomic randomized controlled trial among workers with neck and upper extremity pain. *Occup Environ Med.*

Chapter 16

No references listed.

Chapter 17

No references listed.

Chapter 18

Wassom, D.J., Lyons, K.E., Pahway, R., and Lui, W. (2014). Qigong exercise may improve sleep quality and gait performance in Parkinson's disease: a pilot study. *Int J Neurosci, 1-29.*

Paech, G.M., Ferguson, S.A., Banks, S., Dorrian, J., and Roach, G.D. (2014). The influence of Break Timing on the Sleep Quantity and Quality Fly-in, Fly-out Shiftworkers. *Ind Health.*

Sargent, C., Lastella, M., Halson, S.L., and Roach, G.D. (2014). The impact of training schedules on the sleep and fatigue of elite athletes. *Chronobiol Int. 1-9.*

Liao, F., Zhang, T.J., Mahan, T.E., Jiang, H., and Holtzman, D.M. (2014). Effects of growth hormone-releasing hormone on sleep and brain interstitial fluid amyloid-O in an APP transgenic mouse model. *Brain Behav Immun.*

Kovas, F.M. et al. Patients with Neck Pain are Less Likely to Improve if They Suffer From Poor Sleep Quality. A Prospective Study in Routine Practice. (2014). *Clin J Pain.*

Lusa, S., Miranda, H., Luukkonen, R., and Punakallio, (2014). A. Sleep disturbances predict long-term changes in low back pain among Finnish firefighters: 13-year follow-study. *Int Arch Occup Environ Health.*

Chapter 19

Quilter, D. (2013 June 07). *How Texting Can Give You A Permanent Pain In The Neck.* Retrieved from http://www.forbes.com/sites/nextavenue/2013/06/07/how-texting-cangive-you-a-permanent-pain-in-the-neck/

Chapter 20

Bovenzi, M. A prospective cohort study of neck and shoulder pain in professional drivers. (2014). *Ergonomics.* 1-14.

Noda, M. et al. (2014). Occupational risk factors for low back pain among drivers of three-wheelers in Sri Lanka. *Int J Occup Environ Health.*

Skandfer, M., Talykova, L., Brenn, T. Nilsson, T., and Vaktskjold, A. (2014). Low back pain among mineworkers in relation to driving, cold environment and ergonomics. *Ergonomics.* 1-8.

Chapter 21

Schwecherl, L. (2014 August 6). *21 Low-Impact Workouts That Are More Effective Than You Think.* Retrieved from http://greatist.com/fitness/take-it-easy-21-unexpected-lowimpact-workouts

Chapter 22

Drake, J.D.M., Fischer, S.L, Brown, S.H.M., and Callaghan, J. P.

(2006). Do Exercise Balls Provide a Training Advantage for Trunk Extensor Exercise? A Biomechanical Evaluation. *JMPT 29(5)*, 354-362.

Chapter 23

Hess, J.A. and Woollacott, M. (2005). Effect of High-Intensity Strength-Training on Functional Measures of Balance Ability in Balance-Impaired Older Adults. *JMPT 28(8)*, 582-590.

Hawk, C. and Cambron, J. (2009). Chiropractic Care for Older Adults: Effects on Balance, Dizziness, and Chronic Pain. *JMPT (32)6*, 431-437. doi: 10.1016/j.jmpt.2009.06.009.

Holt, K.R., Haavik, H., and Elley, R.C. (2012). The Effects of Manual Therapy on Balance and Falls: A Systematic Review. *JMPT (35)3*, 227-234.

Freistas, S.R. et al. (2014). Responses to static stretching are dependent on stretch intensity and duration. *Clin Physiol Funct Imaging*. doi: 10.1111/cpf.12186.

Beltrão, N.B., Ritti-Dias, R.M., Pitangui, AC., and De Araújo, R.C. (2014). Correlation between Acute and Short-Term Changes in Flexibility Using Two Stretching Techniques. *Int J Sports Med.*

Gothe, N.P., Kramer, A.F., and McAuley, E. (2014). The effects of an 8-week hatha yoga intervention on executive function in older adults. *J Gerontol A Bio Sci Med Sci 69(9)*, 1109-1116. oi: 10.1093/gerona/glu095.

Freitas, S. et al. Are Rest Intervals Between Stretching Repetitions Effective to Acutely Increase Range of Motion. (2014). *Int J Sports Physiol Perform.*

Kelley, K.K., Aaron, D. Hynds, K., Machado, E. and Wolff, M. The Effects of a Therapeutic Yoga Program on Postural Control, Mobility and Gait Speed in Community-Dwelling Older Adults. *J Altern Complement Med.*

Chapter 24

Gomez-Pinilla, F. Brain foods: the effects of nutrients on brain function. Nat rev *Neurosc Jul 2008*; 9(7), 568-578.

Myles, IA. (2014). Fast food fever: reviewing the impacts of the Western diet on immunity. *Nutritional Journal*, 13(16). doi:10.1186/1475-2891-13-61

Ding, E.L., Hutfless, S.M., Ding, X. and Girotra, S. (2006). Chocolate and Prevention of Cardiovascular Disease: A Systematic Review. *Nutrition Metabolism (3)3, 2.*

Ariefdjoham, M.W. and Savaicino, D.A. (2005). Chocolate and cardiovascular health: is it too good to be true? *Nutrition Reviews 63(12 Pt 1)*, 427-430.

Chapter 25

Author not listed. (2004 February 11). *Dietary Reference Intakes: Water, Potassium, Sodium, Chloride, and Sulfate.* Retrieved from http://www.iom.edu/Reports/2004/Dietary-Reference-Intakes-Water-Potassium-SodiumChloride-and-Sulfate.aspx

Chapter 26

MacMillan, A. (2014). *14 Foods That Fight Inflammation.* Retrieved from http://www.health.com/health/gallery/0,,20705881,00. html

Peng Ho, W. (2013). *Top 10 Inflammatory Foods to Avoid Like the Plague.* Retrieved from http://eatlocalgrown.com/article/ 12131-top-10-inflammatory-foods-to-avoid-likethe-plague. html

Reinberg, S. (2013 March 6). *Processed Meat May Play A Part in Early Death: Study.* Retrieved from http://www.webmd.com/heart-disease/news/20130306/processed-meatmay-play-a-part-in-early-death-study

Kotz, D. (2008 June 23). *Time in the Sun: How Much is Needed for Vitamin D?* Retrieved from http://health.usnews.com/health-news/familyhealth/heart/articles/2008/06/23/time-in-the-sun-how-much-is-needed-for-vitamin-d

Bruso, J. (2014). *The Health Side Effects of Refined Grains.* Retrieved from http://healthyeating.sfgate.com/health-side-effects-refined-grains-3064.html

Nogrady, B. (2013) *The hard facts on food additives.* Retrieved from http://www.abc.net.au/health/features/stories/2013/02/14/3684208.htm

Chapter 27

Author not listed. (Year). *Top 10 Foods Highest in Calcium.* Retrieved from http://www.healthaliciousness.com/articles/foods-high-in-calcium.php

George, J.P, Shobha, R. and Lazarus, F.J. (2013). Folic acid: A positive influence on periodontal tissues during health and disease. *International Journal of Health & Allied Sciences (2)*3, 145-152.

Author not listed. (Year). *Top 10 Foods Highest in Magnesium.* Retrieved from http://www.healthaliciousness.com/articles/foods-high-in-magnesium.php

Author not listed. (Year). *Top 10 Foods Highest in Phosphorus.* Retrieved from http://www.healthaliciousness.com/articles/high-phosphorus-foods.php

Chapter 28

Author not listed. (2008). *Emotions and Health.* Retrieved from http://www.nlm.nih.gov/medlineplus/magazine/issues/winter08/articles/winter08pg4.html

Chapter 29

No references listed.

Chapter 30

No references listed.

Chapter 31

No references listed.

How to Contact the Author

Dr. Tiffany T. Butler is the founder and CEO of Harmonious Living Chiropractic: Fitness & Wellness Center, in Laurel, Maryland. A healthcare center dedicated to providing alternative healthcare services for people who suffer from diseases of the body that is expressed as musculoskeletal complaints. Dr. Butler's approach to helping patients is simple, take care of the person and not the condition, then and only then, will healing begin.

At an early age, Dr. Butler always knew that she would one day become a pediatrician, but her desire to help "sick" people get better without medicine was discovered through chiropractic. Needless to say, she did not attend medical school. With passion and ambition, Dr. Butler received her doctorate from Life University in May 2009. A critical part of Dr. Butler's practice is through community service. She firmly believes in giving back and believes more people would benefit if more healthcare physicians occasionally abandon their offices and get face-to-face with the community. She has held several health workshops throughout the community featuring such topics as Back Pain Prevention and Nutrition.

Dr. Butler welcomes reader response to this book. You can contact her by phone at: (240) 264-6372 or email: info@drtiffanybutler.com. Visit her website for more information, www.drtiffanybutler.com.

Dr. Butler is a workshop presenter and a member of the local Chamber of Commerce. She would be delighted to address your next convention, conference, community group, employees, school or organization.

www.ingramcontent.com/pod-product-compliance
Lightning Source LLC
Chambersburg PA
CBHW070641290526
45790CB00001B/157

* 9 7 8 1 4 8 0 9 2 9 7 1 5 *